Leadership in Movement Disorders

Susanne A. Schneider • Cynthia Comella
Editors

Leadership in Movement Disorders

Expert Advice and Crucial Career Moments

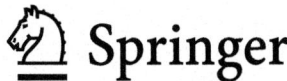 Springer

Editors
Susanne A. Schneider
Department of Neurology
Ludwig-Maximilians-Universität München
Munich, Bayern
Germany

Cynthia Comella
Department of Neurology
Rush University Medical Center
Chicago, IL
USA

ISBN 978-3-030-12966-8   ISBN 978-3-030-12967-5 (eBook)
https://doi.org/10.1007/978-3-030-12967-5

© Springer Nature Switzerland AG 2019
This work is subject to copyright. All rights are reserved by the Publisher, whether the whole or part of the material is concerned, specifically the rights of translation, reprinting, reuse of illustrations, recitation, broadcasting, reproduction on microfilms or in any other physical way, and transmission or information storage and retrieval, electronic adaptation, computer software, or by similar or dissimilar methodology now known or hereafter developed.
The use of general descriptive names, registered names, trademarks, service marks, etc. in this publication does not imply, even in the absence of a specific statement, that such names are exempt from the relevant protective laws and regulations and therefore free for general use.
The publisher, the authors, and the editors are safe to assume that the advice and information in this book are believed to be true and accurate at the date of publication. Neither the publisher nor the authors or the editors give a warranty, expressed or implied, with respect to the material contained herein or for any errors or omissions that may have been made. The publisher remains neutral with regard to jurisdictional claims in published maps and institutional affiliations.

This Springer imprint is published by the registered company Springer Nature Switzerland AG
The registered company address is: Gewerbestrasse 11, 6330 Cham, Switzerland

Preface

Leaders inspire us to go beyond the ordinary and motivate us to move forward to realize a vision. In this collection, we highlight the stories of successful leaders. We are given the opportunity to learn from their accomplishments as well as their mishaps. Although each leader takes a unique path, a common thread runs through many of these stories. The intent of this book is to provide insights into the meaningful milestones of leaders and world experts in the field of movement disorders/neurology. Although we have selected leaders representing only one specialty, many of the lessons learned could be applied to any endeavor, be it an area of neurology or within a society. The individual stories reflect many of the principles of leadership: vision, innovation, building a team, setting the example, and celebrating success. How do they deal with difficult situations? What passion drives them? What makes them a good leader?

Susanne is the driving force behind this book, with Cindy being right behind her. The idea was inspired by a new initiative of the International Parkinson and Movement Disorder Society (MDS), a society that includes more than 8400 specialists. Although the focus of the society is to disseminate knowledge and promote research, the MDS is committed to the new generation. The society fosters a nourishing environment for the leaders of tomorrow through their leadership program. We have been involved in this program and have gone on to teach the elements of leadership to the young members of the MDS. In this process, we have built a strong relationship of trust, inspiration, and friendship with many of the students who have gone on to leadership positions within the MDS and other areas of academic growth.

Let us sit down and listen to some of the best leaders—a fireside chat that goes beyond the clinical clues and science but explores the pearls of wisdom that have helped shape their successful careers. The stories in this book have value that transcends our research society and provide lessons in leadership that have application to so many aspects of our professional and personal lives.

We want to take this opportunity to thank our mentors and the contributors to this book. These are the people who have shaped our lives and the lives of so many others. We dedicate this book to them, our families, our partners, our children, and all of the future leaders.

Munich, Germany   Susanne A. Schneider
Chicago, IL   Cynthia Comella

Contents

1	BERG, Daniela: Kiel/Germany	1
2	BHATIA, Kailash: London/UK	5
3	BHIDAYASIRI, Roongroj: Bangkok/Thailand	9
4	BLOEM, Bastiaan R.: Nijmegen/The Netherlands	15
5	BRESSMAN, Susan: New York/USA	19
6	BURN, David: Newcastle upon Tyne/UK	23
7	CARDOSO, Francisco: Minas Gerais/Brazil	27
8	TAN, Louis CS: Singapore/Singapore	31
9	CHITNIS, Shilpa: Texas/USA	35
10	DEUSCHL, Günther: Kiel/Germany	39
11	ESPAY, Alberto: Ohio/USA	43
12	FAHN, Stanley: New York/USA	47
13	FOX, Susan: Toronto/Canada	51
14	FUNG, Victor: Sydney/Australia	55
15	GERSHANIK, Oscar S.: Buenos Aires/Argentina	61
16	GOETZ, Christopher: Illinois/USA	65
17	GOLDMAN, Jennifer: Illinois/USA	69
18	HALLETT, Mark: Maryland/USA	73
19	JANKOVIC, Joseph: Texas/USA	77
20	JEON, Beomseok (BJ): Seoul/Republic of Korea	83

21	TAN, Eng-King: Singapore/Singapore	87
22	KISHORE, Asha: Kerala/India	91
23	KLEIN, Christine: Luebeck/Germany	95
24	KONING-TIJSSEN, Marina AJ de: Groningen/The Netherlands	99
25	LANG, Anthony: Ontario/Canada	103
26	LITVAN, Irene: California/USA	107
27	MERELLO, Marcelo: Buenos Aires/Argentina	111
28	OBESO, Jose: Madrid/Spain	115
29	OKUBADEJO, Njideka Ulunma: Lagos State/Nigeria	119
30	PAL, Pramod K.: Karnataka/India	123
31	POEWE, Werner: Innsbruck/Austria	127
32	POSTUMA, Ron: Montreal/Canada	131
33	SINGLETON, Andrew: Maryland/USA	135
34	STANDAERT, David G.: Alabama/USA	139
35	STERN, Matthew B.: Pennsylvania/USA	143
36	SUE, Carolyn: Sydney/Australia	147
37	TABRIZI, Sarah J.: London/UK	151
38	TAKAHASHI, Ryosuke: Kyoto/Japan	155
39	TANNER, Caroline: California/USA	157
40	TRENKWALDER, Claudia: Kassel/Germany	161
41	TRUONG, Daniel: California/USA	165
42	VIDAILHET, Marie: Paris/France	169
43	YOUNG, Anne: Massachusetts/USA	173

Chapter 1
BERG, Daniela: Kiel/Germany

It's About the Ones You Care for

Bios Professor Daniela Berg is Chair of the Department of Neurology at the Christian-Albrechts-University of Kiel, Germany and Medical Director of the Clinic of Neurology at the University Hospital of Schleswig-Holstein in Kiel.

Wanting to become a medical doctor since she was 5 years of age she decided to become a neurologist engaged in the care for patients and research in her early residency inspired by Georg Becker, with whom she developed transcranial ultrasound as a diagnostic tool in Parkinson's disease. Her scientific career was motivated by the deep wish to better understand—to better understand pathophysiology and treatment options for diseases but also to better understand the suffering of persons in all the dimensions of life.

After residency she spent two years in a Department of Genetics before she went back to Neurology to lead her own working group and serve as a senior consultant.

Her major research interests are the early and differential diagnosis of neurodegenerative disorders, particularly the detection and validation of risk and biomarkers for diagnosis and progression of Parkinsons's disease and the characterization of specific endophenotypes for this neurodegenerative disorder. The desire to find better treatment options for those affected by Parkinson's disease led her to be PI of many clinical studies. Her scientific contribution to the field can be found in more than 400 peer reviewed manuscripts to which she contributed as author or co-author.

Daniela Berg is deeply convinced that good and sustainable research is only possible in good cooperations. Gratefully she acknowledges many, with whom she could share thoughts, ideas and projects. She is enthusiastically engaged in several task forces of the Movement Disorders Society and in the editorial boards of several scientific journals to enable the spreading of current knowledge. Moreover, she serves patients organizations whenever possible—as it is the patients all the clinical and scientific work aims at.

D. Berg (✉)
Department of Neurology, Christian-Albrechts-University of Kiel, Kiel, Germany

Department of Neurodegeneration, University of Tübingen, Tübingen, Germany
e-mail: Daniela.Berg@uksh.de

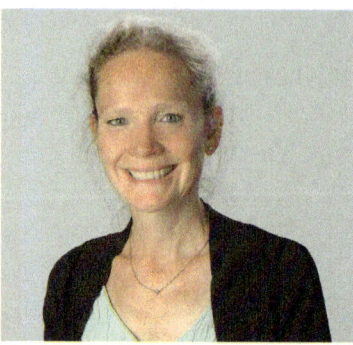

Reproduced with permissions from Prof. Daniela Berg

What was the best advice you ever received in your early/late career?

"Ask him, whether he fears something"—an advice a senior consultant gave me when we visited a patient with malignant brain tumor on our ward round.

I realized that this was the one question I really was not prepared to ask. And this was not because of the fear of the patient but because of my own fears, my fear to be encountered with fears I may not be able to bear, my fear of not being able to give a "proper answer". I asked this question—to this patient and many others thereafter. And I learned that the fears of my patients are very different from my expectations. Many can easily be addressed—once people dare to ask: The fear of pain, the fear of not being able to communicate, the fear of darkness at night etc. I learned that my own expectations and presuppositions hamper my understanding of my patients, in fact of many people I deal with every day—and also of the ones I lead. And I learned to ask honest questions and to endure not being able to have an answer to all the need and suffering I encounter. Most of all, however, I learned that many patients cherish honest questions and are grateful to meet people who are ready to listen to and endure their burden.

What does this mean for your leadership?

As much as I need to understand my patients I need to understand the persons I have the privilege to lead. Before I take a leading position I try to meet some of the people I will be responsible for. I try to understand their situation, their goals, dreams and needs.

When a problem in a team needs to be solved it is first about understanding and then about finding a solution *together*. We all need to be aware that each of us only grasps part of reality.

This attitude is also important for me when I lecture to my students or give a talk at a scientific meeting: It is not about me presenting my knowledge, but about the ones who listen—to give them the best possible way to understand.

How do you measure success for you as a leader?

My success as a leader is mirrored in the success of those, whom I lead. As a *leader in science* a major achievement is seeing those, whom I lead, becoming successful leaders themselves—leaders in specific fields of science as well as role models for others. As a *director of a department of neurology* my success is the generation of excellent neurologists—excellent in clinics, deeply grounded in the integration of all human aspects essential for being a good doctor and knowledgeable in economic and societal issues. As a *university teacher* my success should be seen in highly inspired, deeply interested students, who decide to invest their lives for being a good doctor and scientist.

When do you consider partnering with others, what factors are deal-breakers for you? How do you balance partnership and competition in science?

I am open and teach to be open, to see, whether others may contribute to our projects or whether the persons I lead may contribute to the projects of others to allow new aspects to emerge and accelerate scientific progress. Fair sharing is an integral part of this attitude.

When others cannot adhere to fairness, when they violate the (often unwritten) intellectual property rights or when I realize that specific personalities simply don't match, I quietly quit the partnership.

What is the most difficult part of being a leader?

To keep the priorities one decided for. As a medical doctor in charge of a medical team the most important priority is people: the team itself and patients. As a teacher at university the most important priority is the students. And as a researcher an essential priority is the team and cooperating partners. In each of these fields, there are many distracting factors: economic pressure, political issues, and scientific achievements with all its facets. They all need to be taken seriously and handled diligently. But they should never distract from the utmost priority: care for the ones you lead.

How do you lead through change?

I encourage all to "give it a try"—and I keep saying that problems are an integral component of changes and that new possibilities can only come to life when some old customs and habits die. I try to be ***present*** to see challenges, to listen to problems and to find solutions ***together*** when problems arise.

What advice would you give someone going into a leadership position for the first time?

As a leader one needs to be clear, predictable, fair, and whenever possible calm. Demonstration of power is rather demonstration of inner weakness.

Thus, be modest and honest. You do not need to know everything. But you need to work hard to understand things you do not know.

Be aware that people will look at you—the way you handle questions/problems will be copied.

Always signal that you have time for those who want to talk to you. Especially in the beginning it will be essential to listen and to understand.

And walk up to those, who do not come themselves. You need to understand the people you lead.

Chapter 2
BHATIA, Kailash: London/UK

Bios Professor Kailash P. Bhatia is Professor of Clinical Neurology in the Sobell Department of Movement Neuroscience at the Institute of Neurology, UCL, Queen Square, London, and an Honorary Consultant Neurologist at the affiliated National Hospital for Neurology, Queen Square.

He obtained his basic medical degree and neurology training in Mumbai India and further training in neurogenetics and movement disorders with the late Professors Anita Harding and David Marsden. He is a Fellow of the Royal College of Physicians (FRCP) and corresponding Fellow of the American Academy of Neurology (FAAN).

His main research interest is in merging clinical, electrophysiological, and genetic methods to study the pathophysiology of movement disorders. He has particular interest in genetics of Parkinson's disease, the dystonias, atypical parkinsonism and also rare movement disorders. He has over 500 peer reviewed published articles with a current Google H index of 90. He has also published several book chapters and edited 3 books including a large reference tome "Marsden's book of Movement Disorders" which was the recipient of the best book in Neuroscience award at the BMA awards in 2013.

He is the founding and current Editor of Movement Disorders Clinical Practice Journal (MDCP) having been Associate Editor of the Movement Disorders Journal (MDJ) for over 4 years.

He has had an active leadership role in the International Parkinson's disease and Movement Disorders Society (MDS) which he joined over 20 years ago and has served on various committees of the MDS including the International Executive Committee (IEC) and the Central Science Programme Committee (CSPC). He has been on various task forces of the MDS and recently completed two successful works including the new consensus definition of dystonia (Albanese, Bhatia et al., MDJ 2013) and the CBD and PSP task forces. He has led the tremor classification

---

K. P. Bhatia (✉)
Department of Clinical and Movement Neuroscience, UCL, Institute of Neurology, Queen Square, London, UK
e-mail: k.bhatia@ucl.ac.uk

subcommittee of the MDS and leading to the new International consensus statement on tremor published recently (Bhatia et al., MDJ 2017).

He has enjoyed participating and has been faculty on numerous occasions at the annual meeting of the MDS and has been an invited speaker at various International and National Forums including the AAN, ABN, erstwhile ENS and the current EAN meetings.

He has trained more than 40 research fellows from over 20 different countries, and it is indeed a pleasure for him to see so many of them now extremely successful in the academic forum and assuming leadership roles themselves in the MDS.

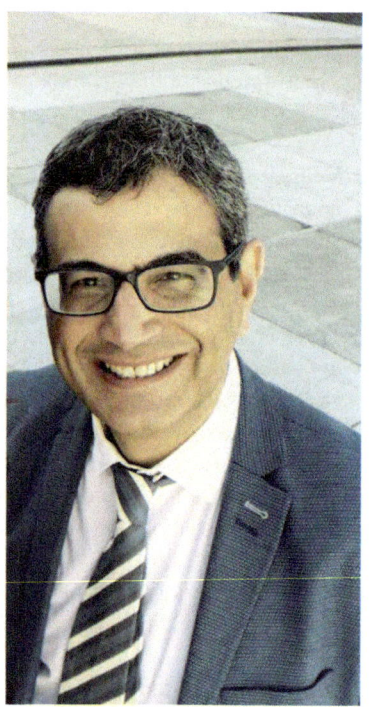

Reproduced with permission from Prof. Kailash P. Bhatia

How did you become a leader in your field?

I actually don't think of myself as a leader in the field, so if I am considered to be one, it must be serendipity. I was lucky to have very good mentorship during my own career with great leaders such as Prof Noshir Wadia, Anita Harding and lastly David Marsden guide me and I suppose one consciously or subconsciously learns and emulate one's mentors. Great leaders are those who can nurture and bring the best in one's juniors and team members. Over the years (just like I received), I trained and nurtured so many fantastic individuals and made opportunities for them to succeed and grow and become leaders themselves. I consider this as my main achievement as a leader.

In your mind, what are the main clues towards a successful career?

I think it's important to have the talent in your chosen area of expertise and then of course one has to be in the right place at the right time and if an opportunity arises one must grab it and make the most of it. So I think the key features are having the talent and getting the opportunity. Having said that however, I do also strongly believe that one creates one's own reality (or opportunities).

Was there any "worst" career advise you ever got?

I did have people whisper to me as I was going up the academic ladder in my career path in the UK, that I should consider going back to India my home country "as there will never be a place for us people of colour" to succeed in this foreign land. I am glad I didn't accept this advice—I believed that there are impediments in everyone's path irrespective of colour or race and it's for the individual to take this as a challenge and succeed nevertheless. I never doubted that I would do reasonably well irrespective of where I was—such insecurity usually stems from doubts in one's own ability. My recently deceased father whom I was very close to and who gave me great advise used to say to me "Look at the mirror daily and smile and say to yourself—"I am fine and everything will be great because I believe in myself—and anyway what's the worst that can happen? Nothing matters so much!" I still do that if I ever feel insecure.

What is one mistake you witness leaders making more frequently than others?

I think the biggest challenge is not to develop a Hubris whereby one feels one is indispensable and irreplaceable. Science and life is by its nature forever moving. One mistake leaders can do is to hang on when their time is over and it important to get the next generations the chance to become leaders themselves. However it's very easy to develop a hubris and a form of hedonistic attitude and forget this.

What would you like to ask other leaders if you get the chance?

I would really like to ask them some of the same questions I have been asked and peruse their answers and see if I can learn from that. I would like to know how other leaders organise themselves, how they use their time more judiciously, how they decide what to delegate and what to do themselves, and most importantly I would like to know what makes them tick. In this latter context I want to know if they have developed other facets outside their work which they find enjoyable and if and how they manage work and play balance. We all have ups and downs and I would like to glean from other leader how they coped with the downs and pulled themselves up.

Chapter 3
BHIDAYASIRI, Roongroj: Bangkok/ Thailand

Bios Professor Bhidayasiri graduated in medicine from Chulalongkorn University, Thailand, in 1994, receiving membership of the Royal College of Physicians of London and Ireland in 1998 and certified by the American Board of Psychiatry and Neurology in 2005. He was awarded the fellowship of the Royal College of Physicians of London in 2008 and the Royal College of Physicians of Ireland in 2010.

Professor Bhidayasiri leads a Parkinson's disease registry in Thailand in collaboration with the Thai Red Cross society, the Ministry of Public Health, Bangkok Metropolitan and the National Health Security Office of Thailand. In addition to his role as a clinician and fellowship program director, his research interest is in data science from objective monitoring and assisted devices in Parkinson's disease. He co-develops devices for tremor and nocturnal monitoring as well as a glove for tremor suppression. His development of an adjustable laser-guided walking stick has been adopted nationwide by the Ministry of Social Development and Human Security of Thailand for patients with freezing of gait.

He serves as the joint editor-in-chief of the Journal of Clinical Movement Disorders and section editor of the journal Parkinsonism and Related Disorders, as well as a writing committee panel member of the American Academy of Neurology on the practice parameters of tardive syndromes. Professor Bhidayasiri is currently a chair-elect of the Asian Oceanic section of the International Movement Disorder Society (MDS).

R. Bhidayasiri (✉)
Department of Medicine, Faculty of Medicine, Chulalongkorn Center of Excellence for Parkinson's Disease and Related Disorders, Chulalongkorn University, Bangkok, Thailand

King Chulalongkorn Memorial Hospital, Thai Red Cross Society, Bangkok, Thailand
e-mail: rbh@chulapd.org; http://www.chulapd.org

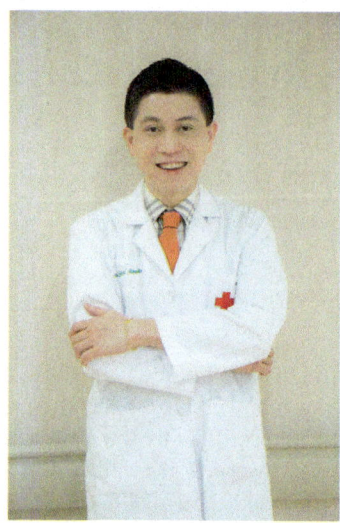

Reprinted with permission from Prof. Roongroj Bhidayasiri

Where do the great ideas come from in your organisation?

As a practicing neurologist in movement disorders, I see a large number of patients face-to-face and, on many occasions, I'm inspired by the resourceful solutions that my patients have devised to overcome their ongoing disabilities with movement disorders. For example, shortly after returning to Thailand back in 2006, a Parkinson's disease (PD) patient walked into my clinic using two walking sticks; one held in his hand as a regular walking aid, but the other placed in front on the floor to act as a visual cue to overcome his problem with freezing of gait (FOG) (Fig. 3.1). This simple solution prompted me to look in-depth into the literature around the use of laser-guided walking sticks for FOG and led me to develop several innovative devices for PD patients with FOG (Fig. 3.1). Our version of the laser-guided walking stick has been adopted nationwide as the instrument for FOG by the Thai Red Cross society and the Ministry of Social Development and Human Security of Thailand (Fig. 3.1).

Another branch of my research originated from a carer's video clip, which depicted the enormous difficulty her husband, a PD patient, encountered whilst turning in bed during the night. While awareness that nocturnal disabilities are common amongst PD patients is increasing, we know that many practicing physicians do not routinely ask about night-time disabilities when reviewing parkinsonian patients and, if they do enquire, patients and their carers are often unable to recall such symptoms accurately. Difficulty in capturing night-time symptoms accurately is probably one of main reasons for the under-recognition of these problems. My interest in objective monitoring has led our team to develop a sensor-based device that is capable of quantifying the severity of nocturnal hypokine-

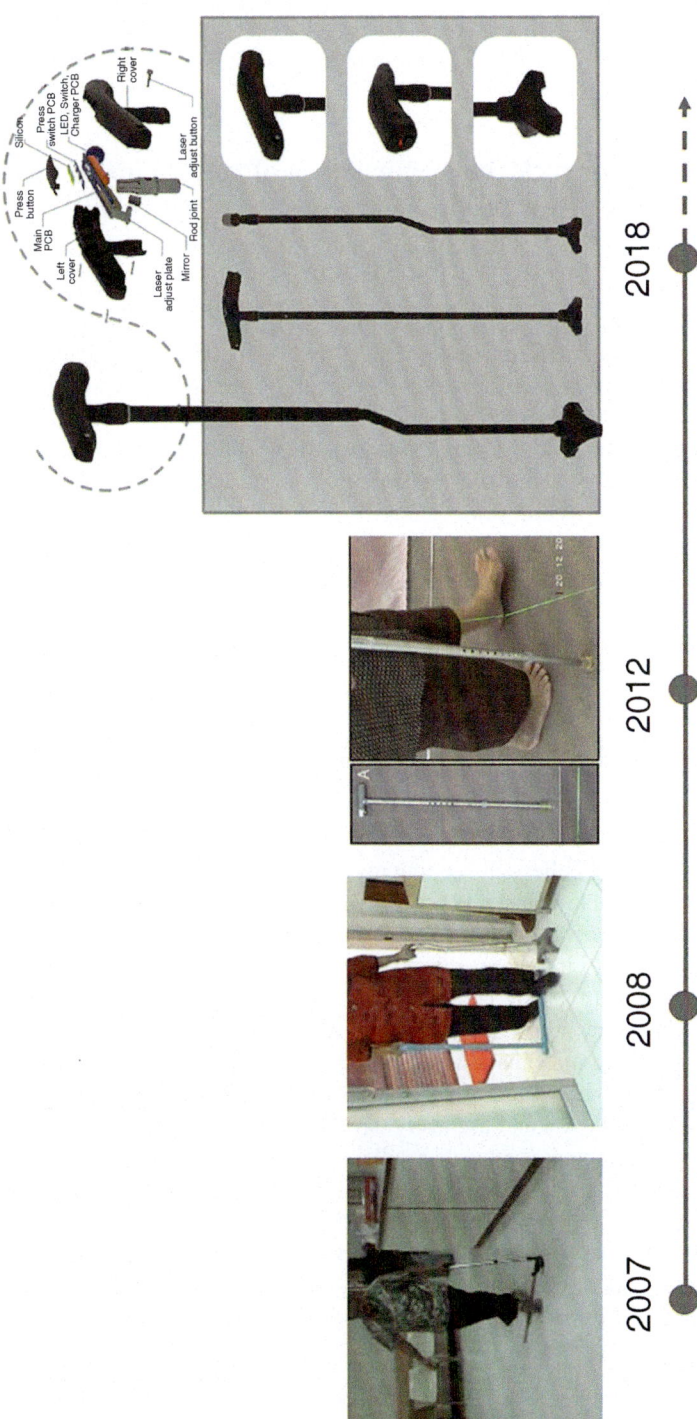

Fig. 3.1 The development of laser-guided walking stick from the original idea posed by Parkinson's disease patient in 2007 to the current version in 2018

sia. The device has already provided measurable outcomes for a number of clinical trials, and hopefully its use will be integrated into future clinical practice.

How would you track the performance of your team members and employees? How do you define and measure their success?

I believe in teamwork that successes must be shared amongst those who are involved in a project. In my philosophy, there is no such thing as a 'One man show' and any contribution, no matter how small, should be acknowledged at least within our team. Success does not come from the effort of just one person, but is dependent upon the work of several people who, when put together in the right way, probably after several trials and errors, combine, like a jigsaw, to achieve a successful outcome. While some endeavours may fail, perseverance is key. Once a sense of 'teamwork' is embedded into a person's psyche, responsibility and application will follow such that performance tracking is likely to become unnecessary as each individual is self-motivated, driven by the desire to be a part of the whole team's success.

What are you doing to ensure you continue to grow and develop as a leader?

First and foremost, I believe in keeping my body and mind healthy, so exercise and good quality sleep take priority in my daily routine. The two books, 'What successful people do before breakfast' by Laura Vanderkam and 'Eat Move Sleep' by Tom Rath, inspired me to transform myself from an owl to a lark and to take regular exercise. Recently, to inspire me to work more effectively, another habit that I have developed is to carry a *nice* leather journal and a *nice* fountain pen with me at all times so I'm able to make handwritten notes, instead of making all my notes electronically. I stress that both stationary pieces must be *nice*, making them a pleasure to carry around with you and use every day. You will be surprised, physically writing your discussion points onto paper will make you become more effective at work, ideas flow more freely as you are less overwhelmed with multi-tasking and you have a better sense of preparedness for meetings.

Last but not least, to be a leader, you need to understand what people want and be an integral part of the team effort. Being open to what other people want and need, and not be driven solely by your own desires, will make you a good leader and well accepted by your peers.

Did you ever consider leaving the career path you were on in order to doing something different (completely or somewhat related)? What influenced you to stay and keep going?

I have NEVER considered leaving my career as it is my overriding passion to work in the field of movement disorders and I consider myself fortunate to have such an opportunity. My interest in neurology and movement disorders was first kindled when I was a senior house officer in one of the London hospitals and I feel incredibly lucky to have found a field in which I continue to feel such fascination so early in my career. One of my patients said, before leaving my office, that she would love to be able to walk like me again, which always reminds me of how fortunate I am to be where I am now, doing what I love. This positive mindset and inner passion helps me get through all the daily stress and obstacles that are part of life.

However, it also feel that it is important to diversify your interests, not by leaving the field you love, but to enable you to grow a deeper understanding. The book 'The design of everyday things' by Don Norman prompted me to appreciate that design is integral to our everyday lives, not just limited to the design of a new monitoring unit or an innovative new shape for a walking stick after more than 50 years of the same design, but also that we can 'design' ourselves, rethinking the way we live, work and play. If you design yourself well, you make your everyday life more enjoyable and satisfying. Then, you can be a better leader with many great ideas, surrounded by an inspired team who enjoy every part of their own careers so much that there will be no need to track their performance at all!

Conflict of Interest Roongroj Bhidayasiri co-owns the patents of the laser-guided walking stick, the NIGHT-Recorder, the tremor analysis algorithm, and the Tremor's glove.

Chapter 4
BLOEM, Bastiaan R.: Nijmegen/The Netherlands

Bios Professor Bastiaan R. Bloem is professor of movement disorders neurology at Radboudumc, Nijmegen, The Netherlands. He received specific training as movement disorders specialist at The Parkinson's Institute, Sunnyvale, California, and the Institute of Neurology, Queen Square, London. He is on the editorial board for several international journals. He has published over 700 publications, including more than 535 peer-reviewed international papers. He also supervised 44 completed PhD dissertations. His H-index is 74 (according to ResearchGate). He is past-president of the International Society for Gait and Postural Research and Officer (secretary-elect) for the International Parkinson and Movement Disorder Society. From 2009–2017, he joined the board of The Netherlands Organisation for Health Research and Development. In 2011, he was elected National Healthcare Hero and Citizen of the Year for Nijmegen in 2012. Since 2017, he has served on the Executive Scientific Advisory Board of The Michael J Fox Foundation. In 2018, he was elected as member of the Royal Holland Society of Sciences and Humanities. In 2018, he won the Tom Isaacs award as recognition of his longstanding achievements in the Parkinson field. In 2018, he was elected as member of the Academia Europaea. In 2002, Professor Bloem founded the Parkinson Centre Nijmegen (recognised since 2005 as centre of excellence). Together with Dr. Marten Munneke, he co-developed ParkinsonNet, an innovative healthcare concept for Parkinson's patients (www.parkinsonnet.nl). Professor Bloem has two main research interests: cerebral compensatory mechanisms, especially for gait and balance; and healthcare innovation, aiming to develop and evaluate patient-centred collaborative care. He also values publishing remarkable observations in single patients.

B. R. Bloem (✉)
Department of Neurology, Radboudumc, Nijmegen, The Netherlands
e-mail: Bas.Bloem@radboudumc.nl

© Springer Nature Switzerland AG 2019
S. A. Schneider, C. Comella (eds.), *Leadership in Movement Disorders*,
https://doi.org/10.1007/978-3-030-12967-5_4

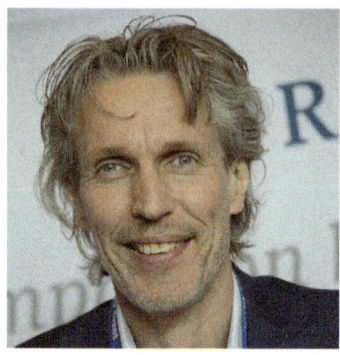

Reprinted with permission from Professor Bastiaan R. Bloem

What are you most proud of with regards to your career achievements and development as a leader?

I am particularly proud of ParkinsonNet, the innovative healthcare concept that we have developed for persons living with Parkinson's disease [1, 2]. It is a new approach to healthcare, where we organize healthcare in networks instead of the usual silos, and with multidisciplinary contributions of multiple different professional disciplines, instead of the usual monodisciplinary approach. All involved professionals have received dedicated Parkinson-specific training, because Parkinson's is way too complex to be left to generalists alone. Additionally, I am pleased with the patient-centred nature of this ParkinsonNet network, and with the various ways in which we have engaged patients as true partners in both care and science. This would be my first main message to young people in the field: develop new concepts not just for, but always in co-creation with people living with Parkinson's disease. And my second advice is to always work in teams, ideally with people who are far more experienced in specific areas than you are. I love working with true experts, and I love bringing them together so they start to create synergy. Another element is that ParkinsonNet is not just innovative, we have been able to extend this from a small initial network in the city of Nijmegen to a now nationwide network in The Netherlands, with branches in the United States, Norway and Luxembourg. So, lesson 3 is: think big, start small, act fast. Finally, a particular strength is the fact that we have been able to scientifically evaluate the merits of this new approach, in a series of large clinical trials that have been published in respected journals [3–6]. Lesson 4 is therefore to always combine innovation with rigorous evaluation. The overall outcome indicates that organizing care within specialized networks leads to better quality of care, fewer disease complications and substantial cost savings for society. Most importantly, this provides hope for the many patients affected by this highly debilitating disease.

Where do you see yourself in the next five years?

I can answer this in two ways. At the professional level, our healthcare innovations are far from complete. Thanks to a large donation, we can now launch the PRIME-PD project (Proactive and Integrated Management and Empowerment in Parkinson's Disease). In this project, we introduce and then evaluate a novel integrated care approach with an emphasis on proactive management and empowerment of both patients and professionals in a real-life experiment in England and The Netherlands. Specifically, this new concept consists of a "home-hub-and-spoke" model with several core elements: *(a)* deployment of extra specialised Parkinson nurses working in the community and who fulfil an important role in coordinating and integrating care and in coaching of patients; *(b)* regional teams including medical specialists and a community-based network of specifically trained allied health therapists; and *(c)* a centre of expertise that supports the Parkinson nurses and regional teams, and where complex patients might be judged if local teams—even with remote support—cannot help the patient. We also perform a scientific evaluation, aiming to provide an evidence basis for the cost-effectiveness of this approach. In specific sub-studies, we will examine the role of technology and "telemedicine" (remote monitoring of patients in their own home environment). At the personal level, I want to further develop myself into a facilitator and coach of colleagues in my team, in particular young people in an earlier stage of their career.

What sort of leader would your team say that you are?

I hope they will say that I am not a traditional leader at all, but rather someone who inspires, who convenes others and who facilitates. My genuine enthusiasm and passion for my work tend to positively affect others in my environment. I suppose my team will say that I am creative, a good writer, and a hard worker.

What kind of criticism you most get?

My team's main critique—and rightly so—is that I travel too much, and one main aim for the next years is to be more visible to my own team. And a price of rapid innovations is that I do not always keep all my colleagues fully up-to-date when new plans or projects arise—this is why we have just initiated a new organisation structure in our group with team leaders who regularly meet as a group to define the joint strategy. Another area for improvement is to keep giving credits to the entire team for everything that we achieve. By virtue of both my character and my posture (2 m tall), I tend to attract the bulk of the attention when we achieve a success, but it is really always a team performance. My goal should always be to put the entire team in the spotlights. This chapter here is another opportunity to emphasise just how extremely proud I am of the many excellent colleagues in my team, and how thankful I am for their contributions over the many years that have led to all of our successes.

How do you get others to accept your ideas?

The strength of our team is to always consider the position of others first. For example, when other countries are interested in working with us to build an international variant of ParkinsonNet there, we do not simply tell them how the system works in The Netherlands, and then try to copy-paste that into the new environment. Instead, we invest deeply in first finding out how care is organized locally, so we know which good elements should be kept (and which can in fact be copied to our own Dutch network), and in finding out which specific challenges are present in that particular country. We then discuss which elements of our Dutch ParkinsonNet approach could be a solution for those specific local challenges. This is a true spirit of collaboration, and even more importantly, it has "learning from differences" at its core—others invariably have as much to offer to us as we have to offer to them. This way, we hope that others accept our ideas because they realize this is a real co-creation. We use a very similar approach in research and other fields where we are active.

References

1. Bloem BR, Munneke M. Revolutionising management of chronic disease: the ParkinsonNet approach. *BMJ*. 2014;**348**:g1838.
2. Bloem BR, Rompen L, Vries NM, Klink A, Munneke M, Jeurissen P. ParkinsonNet: a low-cost health care innovation with a systems approach from The Netherlands. *Health Aff (Millwood)*. 2017;**36**(11):1987–96.
3. Munneke M, Nijkrake MJ, Keus SH, et al. Efficacy of community-based physiotherapy networks for patients with Parkinson's disease: a cluster-randomised trial. *Lancet Neurol*. 2010;**9**:46–54.
4. van der Marck MA, Munneke M, Mulleners W, et al. Integrated multidisciplinary care in Parkinson's disease: a non-randomised, controlled trial (IMPACT). *Lancet Neurol*. 2013;**12**:947–56.
5. Sturkenboom IH, Graff MJ, Hendriks JC, et al. Efficacy of occupational therapy for patients with Parkinson's disease: a randomised controlled trial. *Lancet Neurol*. 2014;**13**:557–66.
6. Ypinga JHL, de Vries NM, Boonen L, et al. Effectiveness and costs of specialised physiotherapy given via ParkinsonNet: a retrospective analysis of medical claims data. *Lancet Neurol*. 2018;**17**(2):153–61.

Chapter 5
BRESSMAN, Susan: New York/USA

Bios Susan Bressman is Professor of Neurology at the Icahn School of Medicine at Mount Sinai, and Co-Director of the Movement Disorders Center at Mount Sinai, New York. Her graduate training was in clinical neurology with a fellowship in movement disorders. Her research focuses on identifying etiologies and disease mechanisms, especially genetic, that underlie dystonia (TORIA, THAP1, GNAL, GCH1, SGCE) and Parkinson's disease (LRRK2, GBA, PARKIN). Her unique contribution has been in helping to create and promote translational teams and her special expertise has been clinical characterization and family studies aimed at identifying relatively homogeneous subgroups likely to share etiologies. As an extension of this work, once genetic etiologies are identified she pursued further translational research aimed at expanding understanding of gene expression; this includes using additional clinical testing, imaging, and biomarkers of pathology.

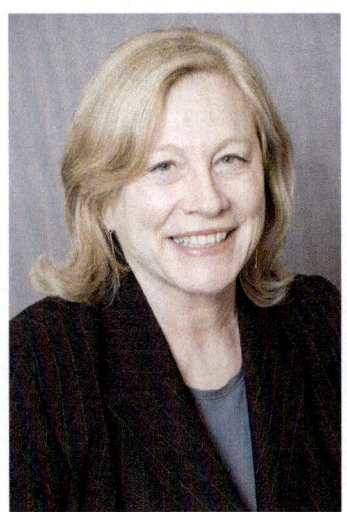

S. Bressman (✉)
Icahn School of Medicine at Mount Sinai, Mount Sinai Downtown, New York, NY, USA
e-mail: Susan.Bressman@mountsinai.org

© Springer Nature Switzerland AG 2019
S. A. Schneider, C. Comella (eds.), *Leadership in Movement Disorders*,
https://doi.org/10.1007/978-3-030-12967-5_5

What was the most difficult leadership decision you have had to make as a leader and how did you come to the decision?

The most difficult decisions for me are the "non" decisions. It is a class of decisions, not a single unique event. I am a doer; I like checking off responsibilities, garnering approval, and saying yes. I also like being decisive. So, saying "no", at least sometimes, is okay too. The toughest decisions are those where I need to decide NOT to act but to wait, and to do that consciously and strategically.

Timing, and patience specifically, is always important—maybe especially in the work of recruitment. Department leaders are judged, at least in part, by how well they recruit. I have tried to grow programs that are well rounded, that promote collegial bonds and productive ends, whether it's research or patient care. This ultimate view needs to integrated into the institutional agenda. US medical school deans and academic leaders look for research growth and research dollars, especially NIH funded which brings both prestige and support to cover indirect costs. They are expecting well—funded research recruits. Then there is faculty practice and hospital leadership. They are expecting growth that is financially remunerative. They want efficient "productive" clinicians. Thus, there are pressures to grow and make that a financial success. Against these growth directives are "facts on the ground". I oversee an established group, some of whom are still building their practice or research portfolio. Adding faculty that may be competitive needs to be done judiciously, ensuring new faculty really adds all around. Also, the faculty you really want may not be ready to move for another year or adequate space may not be available. Often the best path when recruiting, as in other spheres, is to pause, to be patient, and let events and people evolve. The decisions to wait, to forgo what may look like an opportunity, or maneuver around pressures of the moment, are the toughest. I compare it cooking or baking; timing is critical for tasty results.

What was the worst career advice you ever received?

The worst advice was what an official "counsellor" recommended early on in my career. My college and medical school experience spanned the 1970s'. During that decade the percentage of women admitted to medical schools surged from 5% to 25%. I went to an all-women's college. Although I had many wonderful and supportive women teachers and mentors, I was assigned an old school career advisor. I was a philosophy major and although I thoroughly enjoyed my studies, I decided in my junior year that I wanted to be a physician, to help people in a practical way. But to apply to medical school, I had physics and organic chemistry courses I needed to complete. Rather than giving me helpful encouraging advice on summer courses, my career advisor bemoaned the rigorous road ahead. She told me there were many other ways I could help people. Physical or speech therapy were occupations she thought I could pursue that would allow me to marry and have children. They weren't necessarily bad ideas but didn't suit me or my interests. I wasn't thinking about marriage or children at age 21 and wanted to be a doctor. I walked away disheartened and angry. I did not seek her out again, let some time pass, and then networked with other students. I figured out summer courses and happily ended up at Columbia. I learned a lesson I need to relearn all the time. That is: listen to your inner voice and do what you know is right; and when it comes to career, what truly suits you and not what others think you should be doing.

As an organization gets larger there can be a tendency for the institution to dampen the inspiration. How do you keep this from happening?

The key is remaining an attentive and curious listener and observer, to question and not follow rote thinking. For me personally these behaviors are critical in my care of patients and how I use what I learn from patients to inform my translational research. For example, a patient I know for years evolves new problems, new signs, and newly affected family members. I follow this exercise where I treat the patient as if new to me. Start from scratch. Or even if there are no new signs or symptoms, but the patient is one of many with a mystery diagnosis, I need to do the same thing, and then update myself on new genes and pathologies. I am always trying to integrate research into the clinic. Collecting bloods, questionnaires, referring patients for novel imaging or clinical trials elevate care and clinical thinking. These approaches and behaviors help keep me creative and inspired and I do my best to teach this to my residents and fellows. Stay curious, stay creative, and keep asking questions. As a leader I try my best to integrate these traits and behaviors programmatically. Creative thinking includes developing visions for future care, and that can be infectious, even to institutions bogged down with financial imperatives. As a leader it is important to be a good institutional "citizen", but that includes questioning decisions when they appear ill-advised and advancing alternatives. Solving problems, whether it involves a patient or institutional process, can be inspirational.

What are you doing to ensure you continue to grow and develop as a leader?

Years ago when I started as a department chair I attended seminars and read books that informed my thinking about organizational process, leadership characteristics, and health care. I also served on several boards and committees which were especially helpful in teaching me about how organizations articulate and execute their missions, how other leaders and researchers communicate and how consensus is reached (or not). But most of my growth grew out of experience, very hands on direction and management of staff. Most importantly, it grew from problem solving with my department including staff, faculty, and trainees, and hospital and medical school leaders and administrators. And that, along with more mature self-examination (e.g., how and why I react to events and people around me) are helping me continue to grow, in all my roles. I don't see myself so much as a "leader" anymore, but as team builder, moderator, and advisor. Staying informed about clinical and research advances, healthcare directions, and institutional and other department needs are critical to this role. The other piece is working with the team to build our future vision and keeping us on mission. We need to stay unified in our focus on individualized and humanistic patient care, respectful of patients and each other. Finally, there is humor. It is a communication tool that helps me know the group's mood and thinking. There are so many challenges and frustrations, having a leader who can help express the funny and ridiculous side of things helps maintain the team's spirits and camaraderie.

Chapter 6
BURN, David: Newcastle upon Tyne/UK

Bios Professor David Burn took up the position of Pro-Vice Chancellor of the Faculty of Medical Sciences, Newcastle University, UK on the 1st February 2017. Prior to this he was Director of the Faculty's Institute of Neuroscience.

David is also Professor of Movement Disorders Neurology and Honorary Consultant Neurologist for Newcastle upon Tyne Hospitals NHS Foundation Trust. His first degree was at Oxford (Physiological Sciences), returning to his native North East for clinical training and early medical jobs, including neurology. After further neurology training and undertaking research in London (National Hospital for Neurology and Neurosurgery, Queen Square and Hammersmith Hospital) he was appointed as a Consultant Neurologist and Senior Lecturer in Newcastle in 1994.

David's research has focused on dementia associated with Parkinson's. He was previously Director of the Newcastle NIHR Biomedical Research Unit in Lewy body Dementia and National Specialty lead for Neurodegeneration in the NIHR Clinical Research Network. He is a Fellow of the Academy of Medical Sciences and an Emeritus NIHR Senior Investigator, having previously been awarded Senior Investigator status for two consecutive terms. David chairs the NIHR Translational Research Collaboration for Dementia and up until September 2017 was National Clinical Director for Parkinson's UK. He took over as Chair of the Northern Health Science Alliance Board on 1st July 2018. David is also President Elect for the Association of British Neurologists and a Trustee of the Multiple System Atrophy Trust and Parkinson's UK. He has published over 240 articles on movement disorders in peer reviewed journals.

D. Burn (✉)
Faculty of Medical Sciences, Newcastle University, Newcastle upon Tyne, UK
e-mail: david.burn@ncl.ac.uk; https://www.ncl.ac.uk/executive/board/members/DavidBurn.htm

© Springer Nature Switzerland AG 2019
S. A. Schneider, C. Comella (eds.), *Leadership in Movement Disorders*,
https://doi.org/10.1007/978-3-030-12967-5_6

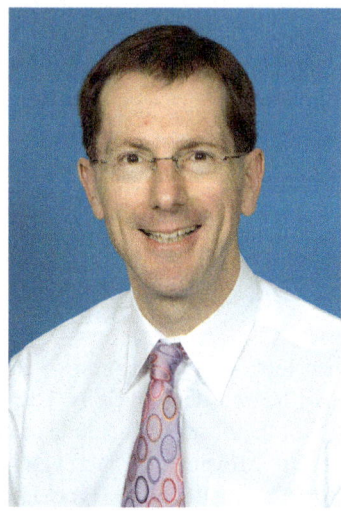

Reprinted with permission from Professor David Burn

Why did you chose Neurology and Movement Disorders as a subspecialty?

When I was a registrar at the Hammersmith Hospital in West London David Brooks gave me the opportunity to become involved in a positron emission tomography (PET) study in twins. One of the twins had Parkinson's while the other was clinically unaffected. I committed to this exciting project, and rapidly started to read everything I could find about Parkinson's and prevailing aetiological ideas. At the same time David Brooks started a movement disorder clinic which I attended as his research fellow, increasing my exposure to Parkinson's and related conditions. I was soon completely hooked! I was particularly attracted to the fact that most diagnoses in movement disorders in the late 1980's were made via clinical skills and acumen. I got on very well with my supervisor, and had huge respect for his academic incisiveness and achievements. I believe good inter-personal chemistry is important to get the most out of what may be your first research experience.

Do remember a life-changing academic experience or clinical encounter? Who inspired you early in your career and why?

I remember several key moments. One was a chance encounter with Andrew Lees at a small meeting in Liverpool where I was presenting some of my old PET work (on glass slides) that inspired me to rekindle a research interest in PSP. I received my first grant from the PSP (Europe) Association, appointed my first (excellent) research fellow, and things started from there. Although I had never worked for Andrew I felt an affinity, perhaps because of our common roots in the North of England. Over the years he has acted as a mentor and been a great sounding board for advice. So from this, although it was never "formalised" with Andrew, I would say connect with people who you can relate to, who work outside your own orbit, and who can provide impartial advice. In other words, establish your own "mentorship network". I would also include my friend Matt Stern in my still active personal mentorship network.

Do you remember a key leadership experience?

One of the most challenging but also rewarding roles I have had to date was as Chair of the Congress Scientific Program Committee (CSPC) of the International Parkinson and Movement Disorder Society (IPMDS). Watching Chris Goetz in action as the preceding chair was incredibly helpful and educational; Chris' legacy of a robust system to formulate the program in far more transparent and equitable way, coupled with a superbly efficient IPMDS secretariat, were huge positives going into the role. As Chair of the CSPC, there were senior colleagues around the table, some with very strong opinions, liberally mixed with more junior colleagues, and those from "fringe" areas of movement disorders who were at risk of feeling marginalised or unheard. One thing I implemented was to treat everyone the same and to give equal value to each colleague's opinion. Additionally, I was determined to keep to schedule and was not averse to cutting the discussion when it was going round in circles on a particular part of the program, or time was running away from us. Neither approach was easy, since I was not the most senior person by some way, but after making one or two telling "hits", the group came (I believe) to respect my chairmanship and evolved into a wonderfully functional and creative unit.

Should a decision maker be right all the time?

"Leaders" do not need to know, or indeed can know, everything. Leadership is as much about connectivity and pulling together those who do have the answers, as it is to create the solutions yourself. Leaders should also not be afraid to admit that they are wrong, or should change their mind if someone else produces a strong and convincing counter-argument. Some see this as a sign of weakness, whereas in truth it is a mark of strength and will ultimately benefit the group, or organisation they are involved with.

What advice would you give a young talented neurologist/ movement disorder expert?

As if it needs stating: When you get your chance, grab it with both hands. I was given an opportunity by Tony Schapira to present on "Depression in Parkinson's" at a UK meeting just as I was getting my Parkinson's research programme started.

This was my first full lecture at a UK Specialist Meeting. I spent more time reading around the subject and preparing my lecture (still with glass slides!) than for any previous talk. It was well received, and subsequently led a couple of years later to a plenary slot at the International Movement Disorder Society Meeting in Rome. Never take a lecturing opportunity lightly; a senior consultant colleague in Newcastle once told me: "You can't make a talk too simple". The related messages that I have always taken from this are two-fold: first, if you don't understand the subject matter yourself, you'll never convey it to an audience and, second, don't use a lecture as an opportunity to show how clever you are because you'll usually come unstuck with someone cleverer than you in the audience, whilst others will just not understand what you are trying to get across.

Chapter 7
CARDOSO, Francisco: Minas Gerais/Brazil

Bios Francisco Cardoso, MD, PhD, FAAN, is a Brazilian neurologist. He finished Medical School in Maceió, his hometown, and did a Residency in Clinical Neurology at the Federal University of Minas Gerais (UFMG), in Belo Horizonte, Brazil. After he returned from a Movement Disorders Fellowship at Baylor College of Medicine, he became faculty at the Department of Internal Medicine—Neurology at UFMG. He is Professor of Neurology and head of the Movement Disorders Unit. In addition to doing clinical work and education of Medical students, residents, fellows and graduate students, he is involved with research in Movement Disorders. His main areas of interest are choreas, epidemiology as well as genetics of movement disorders. He has a longstanding involvement with the International Parkinson and Movement Disorders Society (MDS). He has served in numerous committees, was Secretary of the Society and Chair of the Pan-American Section.

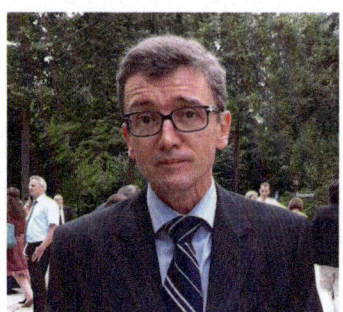

Reprinted with permission from Prof. Francisco Cardoso

F. Cardoso (✉)
Movement Disorders Unit, Neurology Service–Internal Medicine Department,
The Federal University of Minas Gerais, Belo Horizonte, MG, Brazil

What is the most important change that you brought to an organization?

I have been working at the Neurology Unit of the Medical School of the Federal University of Minas Gerais in Belo Horizonte since August of 1993. When I became Chief of the service a few years later, the administrative structure in place since the foundation of the institution had together Neurology and Neurosurgery. This was a consequence of the historical fact that in many areas of Brazil there was no one trained in Neurology. In contrast, training programs in Neurosurgery proliferated in the country at a much earlier time. This led to Neurosurgeons doing Neurology as well. To counteract this was a big challenge because to advocate for the obvious, i.e., autonomy of Neurology was to run into a wall of old standing convictions. Needless to say, this was a difficult political struggle. At the end, though, it paid off. Since the independence of the service, Neurology has flourished both in terms of attracting young talented people as well as in a significant increase of the scientific output.

What is the most difficult part of being a leader?

Obviously, a genuine leader needs to have clear goals she or he wants to pursue. These objectives have to be feasible within the framework of the institution the leader is linked to. Utopias are often beautiful but not rarely they can be destructive as well. Once feasible goals are set, the challenging part is to develop a strategy to bring them into fruition. This requires not spasms of actions but a dogged determination of performing seemingly banal actions over long periods of time. Very frequently there will be long intervals without any obvious result until there is a dawn of a new day where the results become concrete. Another difficult part of this process is the need to deny requests many times made by people are close to the leader. In fact, depending on the structure to say yes might be easy. However, to say no and to keep motivated the recipients of the denial involved with the institution is almost an art form.

How do you set an example to your team members?

In almost all cultures there is a version of the dictum 'do what I do and not what I say'. And indeed, actions are the most effective way of conveying a message and setting an example. Nevertheless, it is necessary more than that. Verbal communication is absolutely mandatory. One of the reasons for such a need is the fact that one given action may be interpreted in different ways by different people. This is more likely so when the deeds are subtle. The leader must state clearly what she or he intends to achieve and spell out the strategy to be pursued. Preferably this must be recorded in written to make sure that the room for misinterpretation is limited to a minimum.

Was there any "worst" career advice you ever got?

This question makes me think about the role mentors played in my career. We know that Odysseus left Mentor in charge of his son Telemachus before he departed for the Trojan War. When the suitors of Penelope attempted to invade the palace of Odysseus, the elderly Mentor was crucial in helping Telemachus defeat his enemies. Similarly, whatever I achieved, it would never have happened without the guidance of my mentors. I can single out all of them who have been decisive throughout the different stages of my career. However, there is an intrinsic tension in the relationship between mentee and mentor. One of the reasons is that mentors are more likely to be more restrained and less adventurous. In contrast, those who are under their wings are often bolder and more willing to take risks. Another issue to be considered is the latent competition often present in this relationship. In retrospect, I do not perceive having ever received a bad or wrong career advice. There were instances though when I felt necessary to act more boldly than had been recommended by my mentors. I do not regret having done this.

Chapter 8
TAN, Louis CS: Singapore/Singapore

Bios Dr. Louis Tan is a Senior Consultant Neurologist and Deputy Director, Research at the National Neuroscience Institute, Singapore. He is also Co-Director of its Parkinson's Disease and Movement Disorders Centre (TTSH campus) and an Adjunct Associate Professor of Duke-NUS Graduate Medical School, Singapore.

He is Treasurer-elect of the *International Parkinson and Movement Disorder Society* and previously served as Chairs of the Education committee and Asian-Oceanian Section of the Society.

Upon graduating from the National University of Singapore and completing his neurology training at Tan Tock Seng Hospital, he underwent a movement disorders fellowship at the Parkinson's Institute in Sunnyvale, California. His areas of specialty and research interests are Parkinson's disease and movement disorders. He is also interested in the interested in the epidemiology, clinical studies and clinical trials in Parkinson's disease and other movement disorders.

L. C. S. Tan (✉)
Department of Neurology, National Neuroscience Institute, Singapore, Singapore

Parkinson's Disease and Movement Disorders Centre, International Centre of Excellence, USA Parkinson Foundation, Singapore, Singapore
e-mail: louis.tan.c.s@singhealth.com.sg

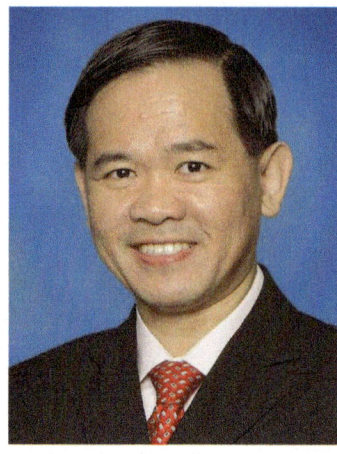

Reprinted with permission from Dr. Louis Tan Chew Seng

How do you communicate the "core values" to your team? How do you ensure your team and its activities are aligned with your "core values"?

It is good to share your core values on a regular basis with the team so that they better understand you and know what you stand for. Beside communication, modelling is essential as people are more likely to follow leaders who lead by example. The core values that I communicate regularly to my team are:

1. Excellence: to do our best for every assigned task.
2. Discipline: to be responsible to follow through on tasks or protocols consistently.
3. Teamwork: to value the strengths and contribution of fellow team members, and to work together towards a common goal.
4. Integrity: to work honestly.

What advice would you give someone going into a leadership position for the first time?

My advice will be to do your best for whatever assignments you receive, to be faithful and responsible to complete them to your best ability. One needs to be willing and bold enough to step forward to be counted. Finally, always persevere and don't give up as long as what you are doing is reasonable, sound, and accomplishes something for the greater good.

Should a decision maker be right all the time?

Has there been a time as a leader when you changed an opinion after acquiring new facts and data. How did you communicate this to your team?

As shared in my leadership journey below, due diligence is important before any decision is made. One has to be open to all inputs from stake holders and experts before a decision is made. The decision made should be based on principles and not on emotions or personal biases. Such decisions should be fair and for the good of all involved. It should preferably be a win-win decision for all, where all or most parties benefit.

Do you remember a life-changing academic experience or clinical encounter?

The 4th Asian Oceanian Parkinson and Movement Disorder Congress (AOPMC), which is a regional Congress of the International Parkinson and Movement Disorders Society that was held Thailand in November 2014 will be remembered as an important leadership journey for me. The meeting had been planned initially to be held in Bangkok, Thailand. Since 2012, there had been much planning and organisation and everything was on track when political unrest struck Thailand with street protest being a regular occurrence Bangkok. This news was broadcast to the rest of the world resulting in many members from the region and the MDS leadership expressing concern about the safety and viability of the Congress. A decision had to be made whether to postpone the meeting, move it to another part of Thailand, or to move it to another country. At that time, I was the Chair of the Asian Oceanian Section (AOS) of the MDS, and Dr. Roongroj (Richard) Bhidayasiri was the Chair of the Congress organising committee. Extensive consultations were made at the various levels of leadership. It was fortunate that at that time two neurologists from Thailand visited my Institute for a short Movement Disorders Fellowship who gave first-hand insight into the local situation and the various options available with regards to political circumstances, safety, costs and other factors. One viable option was to move the meeting to Pattaya, a beach resort located one hour south of Bangkok. The regional leadership agreed. The next challenge was to convince the international Executive Committee (IEC) of the MDS to support the decision. We were fortunate to receive a majority vote to proceed with the meeting in Pattaya. The 4th AOPMC turned out to be a resounding success with more than 800 delegates from more than 30 countries participating. As a result of this, Dr. Bhidayasiri and I were honored to receive the President's Distinguished Service Award in June 2015.

This leadership journey taught me the importance of teamwork and mutual support in corporate leadership; the role of due diligence in making difficult decisions; and the value of resilience in the face of opposition.

Chapter 9
CHITNIS, Shilpa: Texas/USA

Bios Shilpa Chitnis is Professor of Neurology and Neurotherapeutics at UT Southwestern Medical Center in Dallas, Texas. Dr. Chitnis received her medical degree from Grant Medical College in Bombay, India. She completed her PhD in Pharmacology and Residency in Neurology from Tulane University, New Orleans, Louisiana. She completed a Fellowship in Movement Disorders from Louisiana State University (LSU) Medical Center in New Orleans, LA.

Shilpa began her leadership journey as Associate Residency Program Director for the Neurology Residency program with active involvement in Resident training. She started the movement disorders fellowship at UT Southwestern, now in it's 8th year with national reputation. Shilpa helped develop the Neuromodulation network, a multidisciplinary program for Deep Brain Stimulation (DBS) for movement disorders. She has authored and co-edited a handbook of movement disorders published by the Oxford American Neurological Library in 2011 and is currently co-editing a DBS case series book for OUP.

She is a fellow of the American Academy of Neurology (FAAN) and American Neurological Association (FANA). She was elected vice-chair of the AAN movement disorders section in 2015 for a two year term. Shilpa is the co-chair of the committee that oversees the match for movement disorders fellowships in the USA. She is one of the four lead facilitators for the MDS-LEAP program, a leadership program for young neurologists to take on leadership roles within MDS.

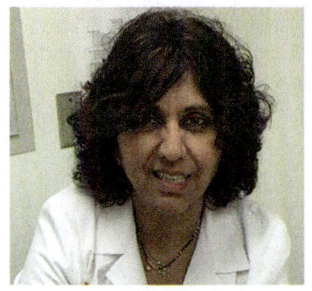

S. Chitnis (✉)
Department of Neurology and Neurotherapeutics, Neurology Clinic, University of Texas Southwestern Medical Center, Dallas, TX, USA
e-mail: Shilpa.chitnis@utsouthwestern.edu

What do you like about managing and leading people?

I never imagined being a leader or manager but this journey has taught me a lot. First of all, when you are managing people, you are actually learning quite a lot, not just about others but also about yourself. Learning from other's perspective, providing meaningful feedback, making changes in processes, seeing meaningful ventures succeed, all contribute to both individual and collective growth. There is nothing more meaningful than "empowering the dreams of others". Life is not just about work and productivity; this journey is also about friendships and creating magical memories. My leadership journey has introduced me to simple, honest, caring and dedicated individuals. I derive true joy and satisfaction from seeing "my people" succeed and living full and meaningful lives. To lead others, I am required to self-reflect and critique and change and grow. Learning to manage people not only makes me a better leader, it also makes me a "better and composite human being"! Growing yourself brings self-recognition and glory but growing others brings with it an opportunity to leave an enduring legacy. A legacy of meaningful partnerships, bodies of great work for others and setting an example for future leaders.

Which is one mistake you witness leaders making more frequently than others?

Everyone wishes that things would run smoothly at all times and no one wants conflict. One of the hardest things to do as a leader is calling someone up on what they are doing wrong or not doing what they are supposed to be doing. Leaders waste a lot of time debating when it would be the appropriate time to have a difficult conversation about deficiencies or lapses. I perceive that if I am doing something wrong albeit unintentionally and no one calls me on it, then they do not care about me. A great leader is required to care about their constituents and by not providing feedback earlier in the game, leaders do more harm than good. Providing timely and meaningful feedback is critical for the growth of an individual. The conversation does not have to be difficult, but it does have to be direct and honest and with an altruistic intent of encouraging the individual to change, improvise and grow in their role and accomplish worthy tasks.

Would you do things differently if you could start over?

As they say, "hindsight is always 20/20"! Insightful reflection of the past and learning from past mistakes is quite worthwhile. I regret not learning electrophysiology and micro-electrode recording (MER) during my fellowship year. I have an intense fear and dislike for "squiggly lines" as I call them. I eventually learnt the skill many years later when I had no choice, as I took over the leadership of the DBS program. As a trainee, it's really important to acquire as many skills as possible; you can always decide later what you want to use or not use. The more skills you have and the more you bring to the table, the more coveted you are.

Another thing I would do differently is crystalizing what my true passions are in academics and not saying "yes" to everything. The "say yes" attitude really endeared me to my colleagues and bosses, but it left me with a lot less time to do what "I" really wanted to do for myself. This resulted in many sleepless nights burning midnight oil to accomplish my tasks. I eventually figured out a balance between wanting to be a team player and helping others, at the same time, fiercely protecting my time to nurture and further my own interests and passions.

What are you doing to ensure you continue to grow and develop as a leader?

There are many facets to the leadership role; excellence, knowledge, dynamism, vision and humanitarism. I have to ensure my credibility in terms of knowledge base and skill set. To be recognized as a leader, I make sure I never stop learning. In addition to reading and keeping up with latest literature, I make it a point to attend a few important national and international meetings in my area of interest each year. My team and I work throughout the year to find interesting things to present at these meetings and to discuss our findings with others and engage their perspective for future research. Teaching is the best form of learning and I spend a lot of time teaching medical students, residents and fellows and delivering Grand Rounds and patient support group talks. I am fortunate to be part of the MDS LEAP course and I read a lot of books related to leadership. I read biographies of renowned leaders, listen to podcasts online and follow the lives of respected leaders. I enjoy Harvard Business Review and the Wharton Leadership newsletters. Last but not the least, I practice my leadership principles every opportunity I get!! Practice, practice, practice, elicit feedback, make changes, and continue to learn and grow is my philosophy of leadership.

Chapter 10
DEUSCHL, Günther: Kiel/Germany

Bios Günther Deuschl had a number of teachers and people to learn from: Excellent clinicians like Albrecht Struppler, Eduard Schenk, Carl-Hermann Lücking; role models like Stan Fahn and David Marsden; good friends, scientists and career-long collaborators like Mark Hallett, Rodger Elble, Werner Poewe and Wolfgang Oertel. He is clinical scientist and was the head of a Neurological Department at a German University with more than 200 employees. He learned the basics how Societies function as a board member of the German and International Societies for Clinical Neurophysiology. He was first trained in academic committees in Freiburg and was teaming in many university committees among them he led the committee for faculty promotion at his University. He published >600 Pubmed-listed papers, H-Factor: >100. He was leading scientific working groups (national and international guideline committees, task forces, scientific interdisciplinary working groups (AG THS)). He has lead two journals among them the Movement Disorder Journal as a co-editor with Chris Goetz. He has led three Societies as a President, the German Society for Neurology, the International Movement Disorder Society and the European Academy of Neurology. Most importantly over the decades, he has collaborated, interacted and enjoyed working with a couple of hundred excellent physicians, scientists and fellows and continues to do this.

G. Deuschl (✉)
Department of Neurology, Universitätsklinikum Schleswig-Holstein, Campus Kiel, Christian-Albrechts-University Kiel, Kiel, Germany
e-mail: g.deuschl@neurologie.uni-kiel.de; Guenther.Deuschl@uksh.de

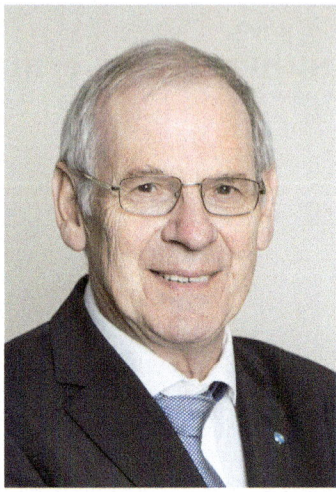

Reprinted with permission from Dr. Günther Deuschl

What is your greatest strength as a leader?

The leader is nothing but a special member of the group and I prefer answering which strengths a leader should have. It is important to have clear aims and to communicate them. Most of these aims are self-evident, but they must be made explicit. Discussing and agreeing on the aims is a major precondition for the successful work as a group. Each member of the group should have its role defined as clear as possible. This also includes that each member of the group must be visible within the team.

Nevertheless, trouble in the group is common and developing skills to bring them down to the aims of the group and the role of the members is an important qualification of a leader. During my career I saw this pattern very frequently, the most frequent accident which may happen is that somebody is misinterpreting her or his role. Then the leader has to find the reason for this, be it structural or personal. Just sticking to the rules usually does not help. Here is where the freestyle of leadership begins: Always keep in mind that every member of a group wants to give his best to achieve the common goal. Understand the hurt toes and do not step on them.

Furthermore, leaders have to be a role model, even in modern days. Never request from your coworkers what you are not willing to do. Also credibility and reliability are key. Machiavelli is not necessarily a role model for scientific working groups.

Finally there is a personal dimension in everybody's self: Leaders often have an early imprinting to get reward from leading a group or a task. Only persons can get good leaders who enjoy working in groups.

It is lonely at the top; increasingly fewer people dare to give honest feedback. How do you seek feedback? Who is your sounding board?

This is true and only few people share their true judgements with you. There is nevertheless a feedback which is reasonably reliable from everybody. This is the non-verbal communication during conversations which tell you a lot. Look at the pupils, the face and the arms and you understand what wants to be said here. Feedback is important but it is also important for the leader to know if she/he is right in what he/she requests.

Beyond this everybody has allies and also few true friends which you can turn to. Also, there is a family which is my personal sounding board for all the mistakes that I have made. I do not discuss the content of decisions but mainly my actions and reactions and having their positive criticism always helps me.

This interaction between you and close friends is perfectly described in Heinrich von Kleist short essay on the 'On the gradual completion of thoughts during speech' (Über die allmähliche Verfertigung der Gedanken beim Reden, https://spiekermann.com/en/wp-content/uploads/2008/11/Kleist_speech_ende.pdf, German and English). He ideally describes a positive sounding board and his thoughts were an eye-opener for me. If this does not help I listen to a beautiful opera.

Have you ever taken or did have to take on a job that you were unqualified for?

This depends on the reason for being unqualified. As a neurologist, there is no excuse to be unqualified and if you have a first-ever situation you have to decide in emergency cases. Otherwise you have to qualify yourself through any medium you can—to become competent.

In science, I found it always important to say 'no' when the project was too far away from what I wanted to research. Here it is very important to follow your personal goals and research aims, because the reward of a scientist is to find good solutions for topics which are of interest for his own reasons. This was why Wilhelm von

Humboldt requested the freedom of science at Universities. It reminds me to the ski ride in a mountain arena with fresh powder snow and getting this right even if there are better skiers than yourself.

If you could go back and give your 21-year old self a valuable piece of advice, what would you say?

Identify your aims and goals. Find your projects. If you are not convinced of a project you should not stick out your head for this. Look for allies for this particular project. The world is not full of competitors it is full of allies. Inner motivation is key: Continue to do the job as long as it is fun and productive. Otherwise make a major change.

Don't forget your family life. This is even more important than the job and remains forever. Try to find a good balance between engaging for your job and your private life.

Chapter 11
ESPAY, Alberto: Ohio/USA

Bios Dr. Alberto J. Espay is Professor and Endowed Chair of the James J. and Joan A. Gardner Center for Parkinson's disease at the University of Cincinnati. He trained in Neurology at Indiana University, in clinical and electrophysiology of Movement Disorders at the University of Toronto (2001–2005), where he earned an MSc in Clinical Epidemiology and Health Care Research. He has published over 200 peer-reviewed research articles and 5 books, including *Common Movement Disorders Pitfalls* (Cambridge, Highly Commended BMA Medical Book Award, 2013). Dr. Espay has received the Dean's Scholar in Clinical Research Award (2006–09), the Dystonia Coalition Career Development Award (2010–2012), and several NIH-funded awards. He has served as Chair of the Movement Disorders Section of the American Academy of Neurology, Associate Editor of Movement Disorders, and in the Executive Committee of the Parkinson Study Group (PSG). He currently serves as Chair of the International Parkinson and Movement Disorders Society (MDS) Technology Task Force and as Secretary-Elect of the Pan-American Section of the MDS. He became honorary member of the Mexican Academy of Neurology in 2008, and received numerous awards including the Cincinnati Business Courier's Health Care Hero Award and the Spanish Society of Neurology's Cotzias Award. His research efforts have focused on the measurement of motor and

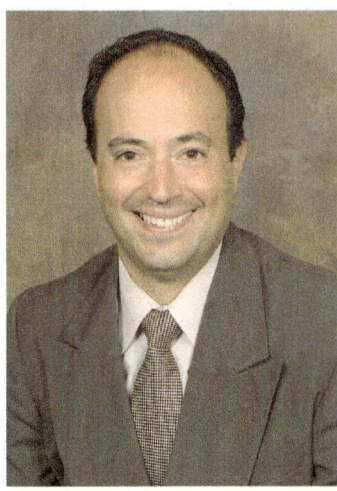

Reprinted with permission from Prof. Alberto J. Espay

behavioral phenomena in, and clinical trials for, Parkinson's disease as well as in the understanding and management of functional movement disorders.

Where do you see yourself and your company in the next five years?

A major metric would be to see my fellows rise to greater heights for the benefit of the many patients that will have the fortune of having them as their doctors. Having bestowed to our people in training the privilege of evaluating all of our patients together has been and will continue to be a source of joy. For our center, the goal in the next five years is to be over the half-time point in our plan to form an inclusive population-based cohort in which to study aging as it relates to neurodegeneration in order to materialize the biomarker-to-phenotype direction of therapeutic development for which we have been advocating. I envision us pushing our field away from the old paradigm of anchoring biomarker validation on clinical diagnoses, which has been the guiding principle of all past and many ongoing studies. On a more global perspective, I see our field of movement disorders fully ending the dominant era of clinico-pathologic convergence for most diseases, proven inadequate as gold-standards on which to validate biomarkers of any utility for precision medicine, and embracing decisively the systems biology divergence that other fields of medicine have embraced already. In this context, we have deliberately designed the Gardner Center for Parkinson's disease and

Movement Disorders in Cincinnati to be an important node in our "collective village" to realize the first of a string of successes in disease modification for future small but well-defined molecular disease subgroups.

What steps do you take to resolve complicated leadership problems?

I get in direct contact with all parties involved in as coordinated a fashion as it is possible. Many vexing issues are, at the core, communication ones. Also, as much as I treasure email, face-to-face communication is most effective in bringing about solutions. It avoids misinterpreted statements and has the capacity to clear the atmosphere from artificial tensions. After any communication gaps are identified, step two is to ensure the problems are not the result of different objectives by the parties involved. If they are, acknowledging them verbally can serve to manage them, much like we do with any other potential conflicts of interest. For instance, in discussions related to hiring faculty for our center, my objective may be to bring someone with unique talents and experience to cover gaps in clinical expertise and research, but others involved in the decision may want to prioritize access to care to reduce waiting times, or looking for ways to lower costs and increase revenue. These different objectives may create tensions that can escalate and remain unclear until a meeting is held. While a single hiring decision cannot satisfy objectives that only overlap in small measure, working as a team to prioritize them serves to realign forces, calibrate the team's expectations, and plan for the future.

How do you deal with failure? When was the last time you faced an unexpected setback? What happened?

Failures have been the source of my greatest lessons and my most important type of springboard for growth. Setbacks have happened both in my clinical practice and as administrator and leader of our center. My approach to both is to gather all the data that can be obtained related to every event prior to the inappropriate decision, or undesirable outcome, with as much detail as possible. Where there rushed decisions? Was there an overlooked sign that should have been considered? More importantly, how could I avoid the same failure again? In addition, mortification needs to happen if the subsequent lessons will be durable. If I didn't feel an ounce of guilt or shame about a failure, then I risk repeating it. The traumatizing pain of a failure can be a driving force to reconfiguring the efforts needed for future successes. Among my most poignant experiences, I always remember a patient I misdiagnosed with a non-treatable disorder who eventually received the appropriate diagnosis and treatment elsewhere. He sent me a letter a few years after he had been virtually cured to let me know about the happy ending to his odyssey after several misadventures, including my evaluation. He ended with a note that reflected I would be last in his list of people he would wish to ever meet again. I felt enormous angst but also gratitude that he had followed up with such important information about his outcome. I contacted him to express both my deepest apologies for the pitfalls unwillingly committed and my humble request to evaluate him again, at no charge, as an opportunity to learn where my decision making had failed me. He declined. After several conversations, highlighting the value of the teaching he could provide, he overcame his reluctance and ended up spending over 2 h with me at the clinic. I reviewed his history and investigations with painstaking detail, and identified several of the signs I overlooked. To this date, many years later, I recall every aspect of his clinical course—and the parts of the history I missed or disregarded became lasting memories, which I have continued to pass on to my fellows. I am surely continuing to make mistakes, but I don't want to repeat the same ones. It is also as much a reminder as it is a source of joy to receive from this same patient an annual Christmas card every December.

How would you track the performance of your team members and employees? How do you define and measure their success?

The first element in defining what each of us should do is based on our center's mission. As our main mission is to help the wellbeing and preserve the safety of our patients, the first question is, over a given period, what did we accomplish in both processes and outcomes that actually helped patients? Our work has greater meaning when it fulfills these core values. Guided by this principle, we make decisions on studies and plan how to track their progress. The deliverables and timeline that we set for each of our clinical and research endeavors are defined from the outset and are reviewed with the full team on a monthly basis until the specific program is completed. How many patients will we evaluate over a given period of time? How are we distributing our work force? Which studies will we prioritize over the next quarter and which we have to put a hold on? We also find ways of ensuring that these goals are realistic and the work toward completing them enjoyable, as much as possible (e.g., can some of the work be done from a coffee shop or even from home, if it makes it easier?). Success is completing our projects in the highest quality manner, with both rigor for the methodology and compassion toward our patients.

Chapter 12
FAHN, Stanley: New York/USA

Bios Stanley Fahn, M.D. is the H. Houston Merritt Professor of Neurology and Director Emeritus of the Center for Parkinson's Disease and Other Movement Disorders at Columbia University Medical Center in New York. His major research interest is in experimental therapeutics, and he has participated in many clinical trials, especially in Parkinson disease (PD). In 1985, he co-founded (with Dr. David Marsden). The Movement Disorder Society and was elected its first president. He was the founding co-editor of the journal *Movement Disorders* for 10 years. He developed the Unified Parkinson's Disease Rating Scale (UPDRS) and co-developed the Tremor Rating Scale and the Fahn-Marsden Dystonia Rating Scale. In 1986, he co-founded (with Dr. Ira Shoulson) the Parkinson Study Group (PSG), a consortium of clinical investigators dedicated to conducting controlled clinical trials on the prevention and treatment of PD. In 2005, Dr. Fahn founded the World Parkinson Coalition and became chief organizer of the first three World Parkinson Congresses in which patients, health workers and scientists review and discuss the latest issues on PD.

He co-organized the first four international dystonia symposia and published the proceedings of those conferences. The American Academy of Neurology (AAN) honored Dr. Fahn with the Wartenberg Award for outstanding clinical research in 1986, the first Movement Disorder Prize for outstanding contributions in this field in 1997, and their A. B. Baker Award for outstanding educator in neurology in 1996. He served as President of the AAN from 2001 to 2003. In 2002, Dr. Fahn was elected a member of the US National Academies. In 2016, he was awarded the Jay Van Andel Award for Outstanding Achievement in Parkinson's Disease Research from the Van Andel Research Institute. He co-authored Principles and Practice of Movement Disorders with Drs. Joseph Jankovic and Mark Hallett. Dr. Fahn continues to be active in patient care, research, and teaching and has trained over 130 movement disorder fellows, including many who are professors of neurology around the globe. Dr. Stan's full CV is also available at

S. Fahn (✉)
Movement Disorder Division, Department of Neurology, Columbia University,
New York, NY, USA
e-mail: sf1@columbia.edu; http://columbianeurology.org/profile/sfahn

http://neuroinstitute.org/docs/Fahn-CV-BIOGRAPHY-AND-BIBLIOGRAPHY2016.pdf. http://columbianeurology.org/education-and-training/fellowship-programs/movement-disorders.

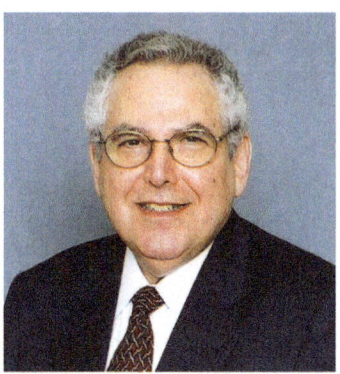

What is your greatest strength as a leader?

I listen to others, trying to learn all sides to a question or problem, and then come to a rationale decision. I think I'm good at analyzing problems in this manner. With this approach, I'm able to convince others about the best way to proceed. Persuading others in this manner brings them to proceed enthusiastically.

It is lonely at the top; increasingly fewer people dare to give honest feedback. How do you seek feedback? Who is your sounding board?

Because people know I'm a good listener and welcome input, I have no problem in people giving me their opinions. Because I try to be fair and rational, people speak freely about concerns or ideas.

What was the biggest risk you have taken in your role as a leader?

I tend to be cautious and not a big risk taker. I'll take a risk if I'm pretty confident the project will succeed. When I conceived the idea for the Aspen Course 29 years ago, my chairman was concerned it will lose money and he didn't want to jeopardize the department and sign off on it as a Columbia CME course. I told him I'll take the risk, and if it loses money, I'll pay for any loss. That forced me to keep expenses low with just three faculty members—Marsden, Jankovic and myself—who I felt could attract an audience. Needless to say, the Course has been overwhelmingly successful and never had a loss in over 28 years.

What would you like to ask other leaders if you get the chance?

Was it your ambition to become a leader? I suspect many people have that desire. Not me. It just came naturally as I became successful in my activities. Leadership just evolved, not from any ambition, other than wanting to contribute to pushing back the frontiers of medical knowledge.

If you could go back and give your 21-year old self a valuable piece of advice, what would you say?

I don't think I would do anything differently. It will be important for you future academic career to have a chairperson who supports your activities and will let you grow. Happiness and satisfaction are related with a supportive chairman. Although I never received such advice, it turned out not to be needed because my chairman, Dr. Lewis P. Rowland was very supportive and encouraged me to do my thing. I was very fortunate.

Chapter 13
FOX, Susan: Toronto/Canada

Bios Dr. Susan H. Fox is Professor of Neurology, University of Toronto and Associate Director of the Movement Disorder clinic, Toronto Western Hospital, University Health Network. She trained in Neurology in the UK and moved to Canada in 2003. She has >20 years' experience in preclinical models of Parkinson's disease and translational studies of novel pharmacological therapies for Parkinson's disease and other movement disorder such as dystonia. She has published over 150 peer reviewed papers, reviews and book chapters in the field and is a regular speaker at national and international conferences. Dr. Fox is Secretary of the International Parkinson and Movement Disorder Society (MDS); an active member of the American Academy of Neurology and an elected member of the American Neurological Association. She is currently co-editor of the MDS website and a member of the MDS evidence based medicine committee on reviews of treatments for movement disorders. She was Fellowship director for the University of Toronto, Division of Neurology (2004–2013) and remains responsible for Fellowship and electives at the Movement Disorder Clinic.

S. H. Fox (✉)
Edmond J Safra Program in Parkinson Disease, Movement Disorder Clinic, Toronto Western Hospital, Toronto, ON, Canada
e-mail: Susan.Fox@uhnresearch.ca

© Springer Nature Switzerland AG 2019
S. A. Schneider, C. Comella (eds.), *Leadership in Movement Disorders*,
https://doi.org/10.1007/978-3-030-12967-5_13

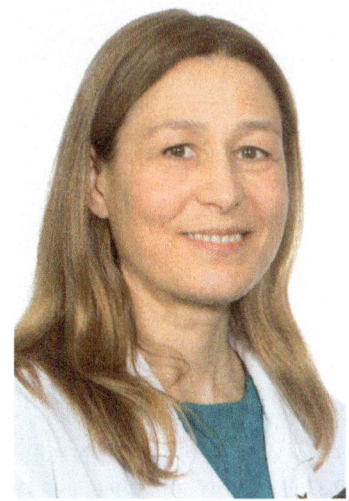

Reprinted with permission from Dr. Susan H. Fox

How do you communicate the "core values" to your team? How do you ensure your team and its activities are aligned with your "core values"?

Leadership by example is the main way to align my core values with that of the team. One of my core values is being thorough—if you are going to do something, then do it properly, don't cut corners. This can range from the simple tasks such as writing clear and detailed patient records with full documentation, to ensuring spending time explaining and listening and answering questions with patients and their families. Keeping to deadlines, not being late or missing appointments, being reliable and giving time to people when they want to talk.

Keeping the lines of communication open is also key—fully explaining what you are doing and why you are doing it in all aspects of your professional life is essential.

Should a decision maker be right all the time? Has there been a time as a leader when you changed an opinion after acquiring new facts and data. How did you communicate this to your team?

You can change your mind but have a reason, and don't switch back and forward according to the prevailing opinion. You still need to be decisive, and sure of your decisions to inspire confidence in your team. However, always listen to your team and colleagues, as they may see things from a different perspective. I have learnt that even if I think there is one way, others may see things differently and putting yourself in someone else's shoes to understand *why* they see something differently is a good way of ensuring success.

Do you have advise addressed to young females in their early career?

Don't be intimidated or afraid to speak up. Your opinion is important and people will listen—If they don't—repeat several times! Don't assume that everyone understands your view—you may simply have to explain it in a different way—so don't be put off.

Having a mentor from an early age is the key to success. Getting someone to speak up for you, advocate and open doors to opportunities is what makes the difference. However, it is then up to you to deliver!

What was the best advice you ever received in your early/late career?

The hardest year is the first year after your training has finished. You are now in charge and fully responsible. However, things do get better! Always ask for help if you need to, at all stages of your career. Just because you are faculty or staff member doesn't mean you know everything. Don't struggle alone. Just as you ask for review of cases as you did as a trainee—discuss cases with your colleagues and peers. Chances are they have seen the case before; "a problem shared is a problem halved".

Chapter 14
FUNG, Victor: Sydney/Australia

Bios I studied Medicine at the University of Sydney. Dr. Ronald Joffe inspired me to enter neurology. He introduced me to Professor John Morris at Westmead Hospital, where I completed my neurology training and then a PhD in the neurophysiology of Parkinson's disease. At Westmead, Professor Con Yiannikas was then running the Clinical and Movement Disorder Neurophysiology sections. He enthusiastically taught me that neurophysiology could be used to interrogate both normal and disordered movement. This provided a way of exploring the link between mind and brain, which has always driven my fascination with neurology. John Morris was a unique teacher—he utilised the Socratic method, asking questions which would lead you to the answers, which inspired enthusiasm and confidence. He was instrumental in providing opportunities for me to become known for my interest in movement disorders even at a junior level in the Australian neurological community. In 1995 John introduced me to Professor Philip Thompson, and I found a generous mentor whose depth of neurological knowledge, both in movement disorders and beyond, but also wisdom as a clinician, scientist and human being, was as great as anyone I know. Philip was instrumental in introducing me to the world of the IPMDS, introducing me to his friends and colleagues who kindly provided me with opportunities to participate in a myriad of MDS activities. The MDS is itself an inspirational organisation within which to work, as it is full of such talented people, and where the leadership is focused on actions and outcomes for the benefit of patients and the neurological community. These activities have led to the additional bonus of the development of many treasured friendships.

V. S. C. Fung (✉)
Movement Disorders Unit, Westmead Hospital & Sydney Medical School,
University of Sydney, Sydney, NSW, Australia
e-mail: victor.fung@sydney.edu.au

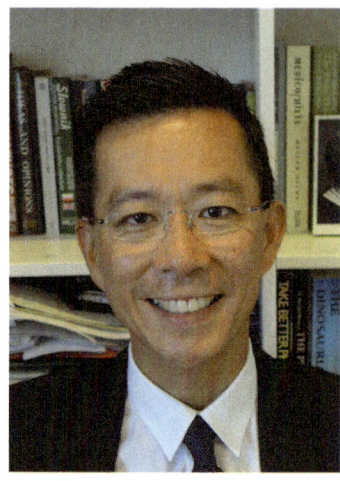

Reproduced with permission from Dr. Victor S. C. Fung

How do you communicate the "core values" to your team? How do you ensure your team and its activities are aligned with your "core values"?

Interesting question! I know that I have "core values", but rarely explicitly state what they are! Perhaps this is because core values are exactly that—part of your core and the way you do things, hopefully good ones and an intrinsic part of your being and the way you conduct yourself in day to day life, not just in the clinic. I believe the core values of a person are not necessarily the "destination signposts" that a person might hold up, but better revealed by the way that a person conducts their journey as they wander between signposts. So, the way that I try to communicate my values to my team is to lead by example, conduct myself in hopefully what is always an honest, kind, ethical and conscientious manner, but also to talk about questions of life and work philosophy over a meal or drink, so we are all aware of each other's values and can learn from each other. Discussing and reflecting upon challenging situations or ethical questions that one experiences, or that are reported in the medical literature or lay press, can also trigger important and enlightening conversations. The strength of the core values of a team and its leader(s) will be reflected in the happiness, success and stability of its members.

What steps do you take to resolve complicated leadership problems?

There are many things that potentially come under the umbrella of "complicated leadership problems". For example, how to resolve a problem where one has a conflicting view with one's own "seniors" if working in a hierarchical arrangement? Or, if one has a senior leadership position, how to resolve conflicting views about an issue by one's colleagues, or how to resolve differences in opinion about the direction in which to take or setting priorities within an organisation.

In general, I try to keep a couple of key principals in mind:

- The problem should be resolved in a manner that fits in with the raison d'être and mission statement of the group or organisation, or if outside of these confines, needs the strong and overwhelming support of its members to change those principals;
- A few core values that should be part of any organisation, such as truthfulness, respect for others, and a humane spirit should not be sacrificed, be it for the benefit of any organisation or individuals.

The first steps are to try to properly understand the facts around a problem, as well as canvas the opinions of others, including representation from both stakeholders and members of the organisation who are not necessarily stakeholders. Open discussion about what needs to be taken into consideration and how the complex issues will be resolved is important, so that there is a greater likelihood of acceptance of the decision-making process and outcome, and trust that it has been decided fairly.

Whenever possible, I try to look for a solution that involves resolution by consensus. However, this does not equate to always simply conceding to the majority, but rather trying to convince the majority to support an outcome that is best for the organisation as well as its members. It is important to be able to identify which things can be changed and which can't, as well as things that must be changed and areas where change is optional.

At whatever level of leadership that I have been asked to assume, the motivation is always to achieve the optimal outcome for the team and organisation, and to ensure that the voices that I am representing are given a fair hearing.

What is your greatest strength as a leader?

This is hard to answer, because of the human tendency for self-deception or affirmation bias! I will therefore answer with some thoughts on leadership and aspirations about the kind of leader that I would like to be, rather than stating what I think are my greatest strengths.

Firstly, the term leadership implies that one is leading, which means that others must want to follow in your direction. It is important therefore, that if one accepts a position of leadership, that one has considered or explicit goals and directions. Those choices need to either reflect the priorities of the people one is leading, or if as a leader one has particular priorities, the stakeholders and organisation need to be convinced and want to go in the same direction. People who find themselves in positions of leadership, but do not have plans for how to help shape or grow an organisation, will end up being poor decision makers, buffeted by the conflicting demands of others and without guiding principles to help maintain course. This first part of the answer about leadership strengths, therefore, links in very much with the answer to the first question above, which reflects upon leading by example. In my view, a strong leader can command the respect and support of those they are leading, because it is obvious that their goals and motivation are for a greater good and inspire cohesion. Importantly, the term used is "leadership", not "pusher-ship"—little will be achieved in the long term if one tries to simply tries to force others to do things.

Secondly, I regard leadership as a responsibility to help guide and look after a group of people within an organisation, not a reward or something to be used for personal gain. I like to work in a non-hierarchical structure, giving people as much autonomy as possible to achieve their maximal potential, helping to guide people so that they find a way of doing so within the constructs of their role in an organisation. One of the key roles of a leader, therefore, is to help facilitate the development of others, helping to create opportunities and to break down barriers through the authority vested in you as a leader, as well as protecting the interests and welfare of those you are leading if they are unfairly threatened. Effective leadership is very much about using the opportunity to advance the causes of both an organisation and as many of its individuals as possible. It is important also to consider all stakeholders, not just those in one's immediate circle.

Was there any "worst" career advice you ever got?

No—so I am going to substitute the below question…

Where do the great ideas come from in your organization?

In my experience, the great ideas in my working life have come from many sources. Probably the most important source of ideas is novel or unexplained observations on or therapeutic challenges posed by patients! Discussions with both senior and junior colleagues from neurology, pre-clinical scientists, or allied health, attending lectures and conferences, reading journals, reading about topics not necessarily related to movement disorders. Often it is an informal discussion over dinner or a drink that leads to the most energising and exciting ideas, and for this reason, I think being part of the fabric of an in-person meeting still cannot be replaced by virtual attendance or lecturing!

One of the most inspiring and encouraging things that I have encountered through my career is the experience that the vast majority of senior colleagues and leaders that I have had the opportunity to meet have been wonderfully humble, and willing to engage in a genuine dialogue with someone less inexperienced or junior such as myself (it is important though to recognise the right circumstances for these conversations!). I think this reflects, in those people, an ongoing curiosity and willingness to continue self-development and consider new ideas, which is part of how they have become role models and leaders, and I try to emulate these characteristics.

Chapter 15
GERSHANIK, Oscar S.: Buenos Aires/Argentina

Bios Oscar Samuel Gershanik graduated from the University of Buenos Aires in 1972 and obtained his neurology training at the French Hospital in Buenos Aires, later on in New York (under Prof. Melvin Yahr) and at the UMDNJ, Robert Woods Johnson Medical School (under Prof. Roger Duvoisin). He is professor of neurology and scientific director at the Institute of Neuroscience, Favaloro University and director of the Laboratory of Experimental Parkinsonism (ININFA-CONICET) in Buenos Aires. He is past-president of the International Parkinson and Movement Disorder Society.

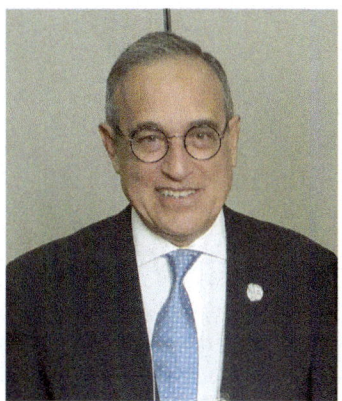

Reprinted with permission from Dr. Oscar Samuel Gershanik

O. S. Gershanik (✉)
Instituto de Neurociencias, and Laboratorio de Parkinson Experimental,
Hospital Universitario Fundacion Favaloro and ININFA-UBA-CONICET,
Buenos Aires, Argentina

In your mind, what are the main clues towards a successful career?

To become successful in your career as a Movement Disorders/Neurology Specialist there are in my view several decisive or critical factors. First we have to clearly define what we mean by achieving a successful career, and in this regard there are several areas or domains in which you can become successful. Personal satisfaction in your clinical and academic accomplishments, recognition by the patients for your care and dedication, and peer recognition of your expertise and scientific achievements. In all of these areas in which we can measure success it is necessary first and above all anything else to be a good person, caring, respectful and attentive; the second factor that I find important is to be passionate and enthusiastic about the things you do, and to love and enjoy your work. No less important is to be intellectually curious, and have an inquisitive mind, and never cease to be surprised by the wonder and complexity of neurobiology. Tackle every challenge in a methodical and systematic way, and be determined and hard working. Gain respect by being respectful of others and by showing that you are trustworthy.

Can you share stories about mistakes, sometimes the best way to learn

Oscar Wilde, the famous playwright once said *"Experience is simply the name we give our mistakes"*, while Alexander Pope the poet recognized that *".....a man should never be ashamed to own he has been in the wrong, which is but saying... that he is wiser today than he was yesterday"*. I will add of my own that those who do nothing are less prone to make mistakes.…..!! Of course I have had my quota of mistakes and always those mistakes entailed a lesson to be learned. My first mistake was very early in my career, during my clinical training. While doing patient rounds in the hospital I failed to uncover the legs of a bedridden stroke patient; my omission precluded me to find signs suggesting the presence of thrombophlebitis. The lesson: always thoroughly examine your patients. Never assume the obvious and apply the rules of the scientific method to your clinical practice, even though the Occam razor principle is a valid approach to scientific reasoning, in medicine, the obvious or the most simple explanation is not necessarily always true. This reminds me of a an advanced Parkinson patient with a 20 year history of the disease who had increasingly frequent falls, which experience tells us is a landmark feature of patients with a disease duration of more than 15 years. Clinical examination failed to reveal additional atypical signs, however, in a routine consultation with an Orthopedist he ordered a spine MRI that uncovered a severe cervical cord compression. The last lesson is to never trust "hearsay". A young man aged 21 was brought to our Tuesday movement disorders clinic by a referring neurologist from another institution. The history and clinical examination was highly suggestive of Wilson's disease, and I would dare say it was absolutely typical. When asked about the laboratory work up and CT scan (there was no MRI at that time) the neurologist told us that copper metabolism and the imaging studies were normal. Puzzled by this I suggested the patient's father to admit him to our hospital and repeat the studies. He was very adamant and asked me to refer him to the best place in the world I could recommend as he was tired of failing to find an answer to his son's problems. I sent him to Mount Sinai Hospital in New York where I had trained. To make a long story short, upon arrival to New York Airport the patient had to be rushed to the Emergency Room at Bellevue Hospital with a profuse haematemesis. The ER doctors immediately diagnosed a ruptured esophageal varicose vein due to liver cirrhosis in the context of Wilson's disease. Laboratory and CT scan subsequently confirmed the diagnosis!!

What are the challenges for a young scientist/academic/clinician today compared to the past and how to tackle them?

I first need to put you into context. I graduated from medical school in 1972, and at that time there were no routine genetic studies, no CT scan, no MRI or complex metabolic or functional imaging studies; the field of Movement Disorders did not exist as such, and our knowledge of the aetiology and pathogenesis of most of the disorders that we take for granted now was elementary. We had to trust in our knowledge of the anatomy of the Nervous System, on the visual recognition of the phenomenology, on a thorough and systematic clinical examination and a proper syndromatic interpretation of the disorders the patients presented with. This trained us to be careful observers, which is a powerful quality for those entering the field of Movement Disorders. The young scientists nowadays have the advantage of having extraordinary resources at their disposal for the study of complex neurological disorders and unlimited access to information thanks to the internet revolution. On the other hand the expansion of knowledge in our field has been so vast that it is almost impossible to keep thoroughly up to date with evolving science and the increasing number of specialized publications reporting on newly diagnosed disorders, new discoveries in the aetiology, pathophysiology and pathogenesis of diseases, new treatments, cutting edge technology, etc. The best way, in my view, to tackle these mounting challenges is to be an avid but selective and critic reader, to attend scientific meetings, to participate in study groups and clinical and scientific rounds, to seek proper mentoring, and to take advantage of all the educational resources available to them. In this sense, the growing presence of the Movement Disorder Society as a premier provider of information and education in our field has been tremendously important. Despite all these advances I am still a firm believer of the power of clinical acumen.

Which is most important to your organization/team: mission, core values or vision?

A tough question indeed, as all these qualities are important for any organization or team work. However, if pressed for providing a single answer, I would say that core values are of paramount importance. We deal with human suffering, and everything we do is intended to provide relief for the sick individual. If we are not respectful of the dignity of the patient as a person, if we are not empathic with his or her suffering we fail one of the basic principles of our Hippocratic oath. The same applies to the interpersonal relationships within our organization. We need to treat others with respect and listen to their opinions if we want to be respected and listened to. Being humble and not self-righteous is the best way to contribute to an atmosphere of freedom and individual and collective productivity.

Chapter 16
GOETZ, Christopher: Illinois/USA

Bios Christopher G. Goetz is Professor of Neurological Sciences and Pharmacology at Rush University Medical Center in Chicago and serves as Director of the Movement Disorders program and Director of the Rush Parkinson's Foundation Research Center. He is the current President of the International Parkinson and Movement Disorder Society. He has published over 450 peer-reviewed articles, over 200 book chapters, and fourteen books. He has been co-editor-in-chief of the *Movement Disorders* journal, and editor-in-chief of *Clinical Neuropharmacology*.

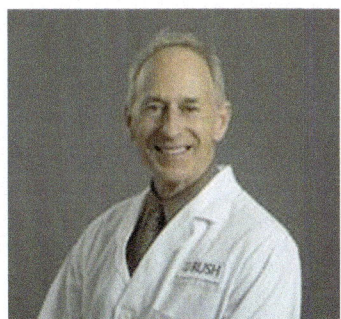

Reprinted with permission from Prof. Christopher G. Goetz

Who inspires you and why?

I have been inspired by my early clinical teachers, specifically Harold L. Klawans, C. David Marsden, Stanley Fahn, and Roger Duvoisin. They individually and collectively taught me the richness of movement disorders as a field of study,

---

C. G. Goetz (✉)
Rush University Medical Center, Chicago, IL, USA

International Parkinson and Movement Disorder Society (2017–2019),
Milwaukee, WI, USA
e-mail: Christopher_Goetz@rush.edu

© Springer Nature Switzerland AG 2019
S. A. Schneider, C. Comella (eds.), *Leadership in Movement Disorders*,
https://doi.org/10.1007/978-3-030-12967-5_16

challenged me to meet the highest level of my potential, and shared their warmth and inclusiveness. Having them with me in my early career to encourage and guide me was particularly important, because a correction or complement from them set me immediately on a clearer path of development. Even today, I still turn to Stanley Fahn for counsel, and a very short exchange with him provides me with guidance and clarity.

Historically, I have been most inspired by the French neurologist of the nineteenth century, Jean-Martin Charcot (1825–1893). As the leading clinical neurologist of his era, he established the nosology of neurology that remains largely unaltered today, anchoring neurology in the correlation between specific neurological signs and their anatomical bases. His contributions to neurology and specifically movement disorders are numerous, but, his reflections on clinical medicine and the role of a physician are most important to me and resonate on a daily basis.

What are the challenges for a young scientist/academic clinician today compared to the past?

Young colleagues have often asked how they can succeed when there are so many peers vying for success. The competition they fear, however, is not fundamentally different than when I was rising in the field, and, in my view, the same steps needed in my era of advancement still solidly apply.

Young investigators are faced today with an enormous array of choices, whereas those of my era were simpler and less creative, either academics or clinical practice. Careers in Industry or Medical-legal consultation were largely scorned, start-up companies did not exist, and Life-Work balance prioritizations were at their most fastigial level of development. A cultural evolution has created a message that "I can do everything", causing, in my view, a great liberation of thought, but also a dangerous edge of poor focus and a serious risk to a dedicated path of excellence. The young investigator who has the needed focus, determination, and commitment to a slow and continual climb towards excellence is, in fact, a member of a very small group, probably no larger than during my era of development. Indeed, there are more people in the field than when I started, but the road has not changed, and the number of serious investigators traveling it while watching their colleagues veer onto the multiple paths that now exist as other options, is still quite small.

How did mentorship influence your career?

One necessary key to success is mentorship, and I was indeed very fortunate to have the very best of teachers: Harold Klawans, Stanley Fahn, C. David Marsden, and Roger Duvoisin in the clinical realm and Jacques Glowinski and Michel Hamon in the laboratory. Such access at the very beginning of my career placed me in an environment of discipline, encouragement, correction, and opportunity. These contacts were entirely self-initiated and highly dependent on where one trained and whom one knew. At that time, there were no organized programs to foster leadership training and growth within national or international societies. Today, both the American Academy of Neurology and the International Parkinson and Movement Disorder Society (IPMDS) fulfill this role, opening up the ranks of leadership training to people with or without direct mentorship at their local institutions. At the IPMDS, the Summer Schools and LEAP program allow ambitious young investigators to access world leaders and develop mentorship models even if their local mentorship opportunities are limited. Personal mentorship is still the core ingredient to success, but access to that mentorship has expanded broadly with a focus on inclusiveness.

If you could go back and give your 21-year old self a valuable piece of advice, what would you say?

- Have the self-confidence and humility to ask for a chance. If there is a role you would like to take, write to the leader and offer your services. Have the perseverance to ask twice or three times, if the first request is not successful. The road being pursued is a long one.
- Choose an area to study that really interests you, since the path is lonely, and you will need to endure more than a few rejections, set-backs, and failures. Be brave enough to turn away from bad opportunities, but stick with the ideas and interests that fascinate you.
- If you have the good fortune to find a friend in the midst of your career, cultivate that friendship with priority, since a good colleague is a cherished companion during a long academic career. Many speak of competition as a threat to friendship, but if one is competing only with oneself and one's own image of full potential, friendship can develop. It requires time and commitment in good years and bad years, can be threatened by the pressures of time and distance, but the fruits are rich and enduring.

Chapter 17
GOLDMAN, Jennifer: Illinois/USA

Bios Jennifer G. Goldman, MD, MS, FAAN, FANA is a Movement Disorders neurologist with specialty board certification in Behavioral Neurology and Neuropsychiatry. Dr. Goldman is the Section Chief for Parkinson's Disease and Movement Disorders Rehabilitation at the Shirley Ryan AbilityLab (formerly Rehabilitation Institute of Chicago) and Professor of Physical Medicine and Rehabilitation and Neurology at Northwestern University Feinberg School of Medicine in Chicago. From 2004–2018, Dr. Goldman was on the faculty at Rush University, Section of Parkinson's Disease and Movement Disorders and promoted through the academic ranks to Professor of Neurological Sciences. At Rush, she founded and directed the Integrated Cognitive Behavioral Movement Disorders program, a comprehensive, interdisciplinary clinic and directed the Lewy Body Dementia Association Research Center of Excellence and Huntington's Disease Society of America Center of Excellence. Dr. Goldman has been a leader in the field of neuropsychiatric issues in Parkinson's disease (PD), with research contributions regarding clinical features, neuroimaging, and biomarkers of PD mild cognitive impairment, dementia, and psychosis. She serves on the *Movement Disorders* journal Editorial Board, the MDS Leadership (LEAP) Task Force and as MDS LEAP faculty, the MDS Task Forces for PD-MCI, Integrated and Interdisciplinary care, and Rating Scales, and the American Academy of Neurology (AAN) Women in Leadership Committee. Dr. Goldman chairs the MDS Pan-American Section Education Committee and the AAN Movement Disorders Section.

J. G. Goldman (✉)
Parkinson's Disease and Movement Disorders at the Shirley Ryan AbilityLab,
Departments of Physical Medicine and Rehabilitation and Neurology,
Northwestern University Feinberg School of Medicine, Chicago, IL, USA

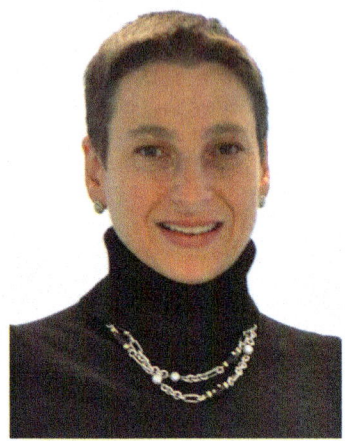

What was the best advice you ever received in your career?

Although difficult to pick the "best" advice, one salient example comes to mind, especially as it comes not from a physician, scientist, or mentor per se, but rather from a French chef. "Nothing is ever wasted, whether in the kitchen, or in life." While much more poetically stated by him, the idea that you can fully utilize, must utilize, and thereby, think creatively to utilize every ingredient in its entirety opens up doors for many delicious opportunities, whether in the kitchen or in life. In my career, I have learned valuable leadership and communication skills from serving as the orchestral concertmaster and playing chamber music over the years. I have developed a solid foundation from my fellowship days in a genetics lab, even though this did not become a primary road in my career. Furthermore, I have discovered that many influential experiences in college, medical school, or even earlier in neuropsychology and neurorehabilitation continuously shape my career, lending themselves to new ideas, new approaches, and new chapters.

What does neurology mean to you?

A fascinating field and a lifelong journey… Several personal and professional experiences, even at an early age, sparked my intrigue with Neurology. Early excitement came from reading Sacks and Luria, playing with neuropsychological "games," witnessing the "decade of the brain," and later studying the intersection of music and the brain and visual perception in college. Trying to understand how the brain and nervous system work; how we behave, think and move in both health and disease; and how we can modify these actions and abilities through medications, surgery, or non-pharmacological ways ultimately led me to focus my career in Neurology on movement disorders and especially their relationship to cognition and behavior. To me, as a clinician-researcher-educator, Neurology remains a dynamic and exciting field, with many questions awaiting to be solved and advancing therapeutics in evolution, and a wonderful opportunity to greatly impact the lives of those affected by movement disorders.

What are a few resources you would recommend to someone looking to gain insight into becoming a better leader?

Many resources surround us, constantly and abundantly. Sometimes they are obvious and specific like a book or course on leadership skills (e.g., classics like Kouzes and Posner's The Leadership Challenge or Harvard Business Review), but often they are experiential and reflective such as the conversations we have over coffee or at poster sessions, or the observations we make of other people's behaviors (both good and bad examples and by those with or without clearly defined "leadership" titles), or when we face a challenging situation without a clear roadmap. My recommendation would be to always be experiencing, observing, inquiring, meeting, reading, and living—whether related to medicine or not. These are the best resources for one's personal growth and journey to become a better leader. Seek it out and soak it up!

Would you do things differently if you had to start over?

My short answer…no!

Chapter 18
HALLETT, Mark: Maryland/USA

Bios Dr. Mark Hallett obtained his M.D. at Harvard University and trained in neurology at Massachusetts General Hospital and in neurophysiology at the National Institutes of Health and at the Institute of Psychiatry in London. From 1976 to 1984, he was the Chief of the Clinical Neurophysiology Laboratory at the Brigham and Women's Hospital and rose to Associate Professor of Neurology at Harvard Medical School. From 1984, he has been at the National Institute of Neurological Disorders and Stroke (NINDS) where he serves as Chief of the Human Motor Control Section and pursues research on the physiology of human movement disorders and other problems of motor control. He also served as Clinical Director of NINDS until July 2000. He is past President of the International Parkinson and Movement Disorder Society, the American Association of Neuromuscular and Electrodiagnostic Medicine, and the International Federation of Clinical Neurophysiology. He served as Vice-president of the American Academy of Neurology. He was Editor in Chief of Clinical Neurophysiology and Associate Editor of Brain.

M. Hallett (✉)
Human Motor Control Section, NINDS, NIH, Bethesda, MD, USA
e-mail: hallettm@ninds.nih.gov; http://intra.ninds.nih.gov/Lab.asp?Org_ID=72

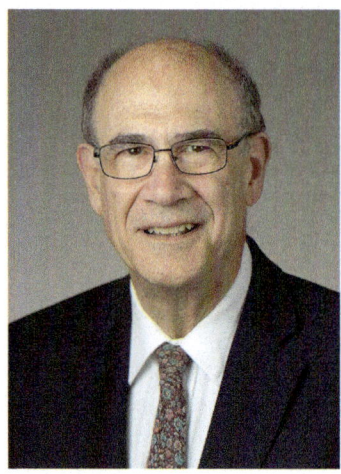

Reprinted with permission from Dr. Mark Hallett

What advice would you give a young talented neurologist/ movement disorder expert?

People should do what they enjoy doing.

There are plenty of movement disorder patients, they are interesting and fun to treat. Often the doctor can help the patient. Hence, straight clinical work can be a good choice. Basic knowledge and therapeutic options in movement disorders are advancing rapidly so it is important to keep up to date.

For those neurologists interested in research, there are two broad pathways, clinical or basic research. Again, the right way is what is appealing. Clinical research keeps you near the patients and is less schizophrenic. Clinical research itself is further divided into understanding disease and treatment. The area of clinical trials is growing rapidly and can be a good choice. The skills needed are becoming more complex, including clinical trial design and statistics, but the rewards are often good. Basic neuroscience is equally exciting; I enjoy working out the physiology of the brain. One way or the other, it is stimulating to be at the forefront of understanding new aspects of neuroscience, as understanding disease can also lead to the development of new therapies.

Certain areas are hot from time to time. These are often exciting since lots of people work in the area, advances can be rapid, and grant money might be more plentiful. For example, in recent years, genetics, focusing on finding mutations relevant to disease, has been very popular. While it remains so, the hot areas rising are epigenetics and cell biology focused on how genes work and how their mutations lead to disease. The most success is for those people who can stay ahead of the curve. One downside is that there is much competition (e.g., for grants) and life can be stressful.

Bottom line, to end where I began, the idea is to have fun.

Why did you chose Neurology and Movement Disorders as a subspecialty?

I developed my interest in the brain during high school. I had an excellent teacher in a psychology class. I learned about how the brain functions and its mysteries. I wrote a final paper on Freud's theories (which curiously I am now revisiting with my interest in functional movement disorders). I continued my interest in Harvard college by taking physiological psychology and neuroscience courses. Once I heard a lecture by Norman Geschwind on Alexia Without Agraphia. He was an exciting and dynamic lecturer. I remember leaving the lecture hall being certain that I had made a good decision to go to medical school and to study the brain. Neurology was my choice.

At that time there was the Vietnam war, and there was a mandatory doctor draft. However, better than to go to Vietnam was the option of going to the National Institutes of Health. I got a telegram near the end of my internship telling me that I had been selected to go to the NIH. There I encountered Mahlon DeLong who studied the basal ganglia. I developed a definite interest in motor control at that time. Eventually, my wife and I wanted to spend a year abroad, and I had the opportunity to work in the young neurology department and research laboratory of C. David Marsden in London. I was impressed with his work.

So really, I just fell into motor control and, then, movement disorders almost by chance.

It is lonely at the top; increasingly fewer people dare to give honest feedback. How do you seek feedback? Who is your sounding board?

To a large extent I disagree with the premise. I work in the academic environment, and perhaps a fortunate one in this regard. In research, at least, we cannot escape feedback. To get grants, we have to compete for funding. To publish a paper, it must undergo peer review. These are both anonymous procedures and this might "loosen the tongue," but feedback can be quite rigorous. Additionally, in my workplace, my whole research program is reviewed in detail by outside reviewers every four years. Of course, the march of science is the ultimate feedback, demonstrating whether your results survive the test of time.

In relation to patient care, I see most of my patients together with fellows, residents, and students. They have not been shy giving alternate opinions, at least in regard to diagnosis. In this circumstance, the laboratory results and follow-up visits are the feedback.

As to issues of group management, I can see how this might be a problem in some situations, but at least in my situation, I cannot be too authoritarian. Too many peers and bosses for that. A collegial environment helps, and it is good to be collegial. It is not lonely where I sit.

What is the most difficult part of being a leader?

For me the most difficult part is balancing management. There is micromanagement on one end and lack of supervision on the other. Where to find the right balance? Making all the decisions and watching everyone carefully would hopefully lead to processes and results done in the "best" way—"best" meaning the way you would want. On the other hand, I believe good leadership allows subordinates the opportunity to make decisions and operate independently. This might lead to errors or outcomes that are not desirable. In any event, as an organization gets bigger, as the number of persons supervised gets larger, it becomes less possible to micromanage. A larger organization makes it possible to get more work done, but being "out of control" is the consequence. There is always some ability to balance the amount of control exerted, so there are always some decisions to be made. Giving up some supervision is not all together bad (since it gives subordinates some freedom), but, in the end, as leader, you are ultimately responsible for all outcomes. Taking the responsibility, when you might not be actually responsible for the proximate action, can be very difficult.

Chapter 19
JANKOVIC, Joseph: Texas/USA

Lessons I Have Learned

Bios Dr. Jankovic trained at Baylor College of Medicine, Houston, and at Neurological Institute, Columbia University, New York City. In 1977 he founded and has since directed the Parkinson's Disease Center and Movement Disorders Clinic at Baylor College, which has been designated as a "Center of Excellence" by the Parkinson's Foundation, Huntington Disease Association of America, and Tourette Association of America. He holds the endowed Distinguished Chair in Movement Disorders.

He is one of the founders of the International Parkinson and Movement Disorder Society and served as its third president in 1994. He was principal investigator in over hundred clinical trials and his pioneering research on drugs for movement disorders has led to their approval by the United States Food and Drug Administration. He published over 1,200 original articles and chapters, and authored or co-edited over 50 books. In 1991 he co-founded the annual course "A Comprehensive Review of Movement Disorders", in Aspen, Colorado, still the most comprehensive course for fellows and other physicians. Dr. Jankovic is current or past member of many editorial and scientific advisory boards of national and international foundations, including Dystonia Medical Research Foundation, International Essential Tremor Foundation, Tourette Association of America, and has served on the executive scientific advisory board of the Michael J. Fox Foundation for Parkinson's Research. He has trained hundreds of physicians and researchers, many of whom have become internationally recognized leaders in the field of movement disorders.

J. Jankovic (✉)
Department of Neurology, Parkinson's Disease Center and Movement Disorders Clinic, Baylor College of Medicine, Houston, TX, USA
e-mail: josephj@bcm.edu; http://www.jankovic.org

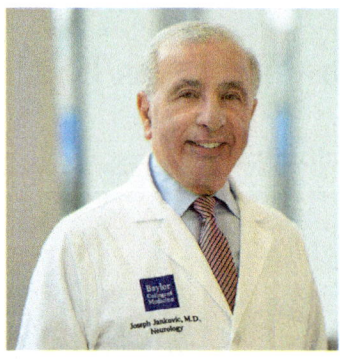

Reprinted with permission from Professor Joseph Jankovic

Why did you chose Neurology and Movement Disorders as a subspecialty?

During my Neurology Residency at Columbia University, New York (1974–77) I was very much inspired and influenced by Bud Rowland, MD, who was the Chairman of the Department of Neurology and a world renowned neuromuscular expert. He became my mentor and a friend, but also a role model how to be an effective, fair, and engaging leader and how to instill curiosity and integrity in students and other trainees.

I later, however, met Dr. Fahn and was infected by his enthusiasm for the field of movement disorders, so I soon also became hooked. I was fascinated by the wide expression and rich phenomenology of hypokinetic and hyperkinetic movement disorders. When I finally decided to pursue movement disorders as my professional career I made an appointment with Dr. Rowland to let him know that I wanted to become a movement disorders rather than neuromuscular specialist. He looked at me and in his typical, provocative but kind and humorous manner and said "You want to go into Parkinson's disease? Are you kidding? You will make the diagnosis in the first minute and what are you going to do for the rest of the hour?"

Dr. Fahn, whom I consider one of my most influential mentors, taught me to appreciate all the subtleties and recognize phenomenological patterns that are critical in the differential diagnosis of various movement disorders. I believe that because of the important role of phenomenology, movement disorders will remain as perhaps the last discipline in medicine that will still require careful observation and examination of the patients rather than relying on imaging, neurophysiologic, or other diagnostic tests. Even during my early training, I appreciated movement disorders as one of the most therapeutically oriented specialties in neurology. And this was before tetrabenazine and botulinum toxin, and before deep brain stimulation. I am proud to play a role in the development of these and other therapeutic advances [1–3].

What is your definition of leadership, what does leadership mean to you?

Leadership may be defined as a personal quality that allows an individual to influence or inspire other people to organize and harmonize behind a common goal so its objectives can be accomplished efficiently, cohesively and appropriately. Leaders must be able to work effectively with people who think differently and be able to resolve conflicts. A leader is like a symphony conductor, making sure that instruments that sound differently and uniquely harmonize into a meaningful melody. A leader should inspire empathy, professionalism and conscientiousness, the most important ingredients to becoming a successful physician [4, 5]. There is no single formula for successful leadership, but an effective leader should also be a mentor for his younger followers. During my presentations about mentorship, I often emphasize that selecting the right mentor is probably the most critical decision in young physician's or scientist's career. An ideal mentor should not be a "tormentor". The reader is also invited to review other relevant articles on leadership and training in Neurology [6, 7]. Although I learned on the job, there are now many leadership programs such as LEAP of the International Movement Disorders Society, American Academy of Neurology Emerging Leaders Forum, and many others.

What are the challenges for a young scientist/academic clinician today compared to the past and how to tackle them?

One of the most difficult decisions I had to make was between clinical or basic science research as I was fascinated by both. While the concept of a physician scientist is a noble goal, it has become increasingly difficult to achieve it and, unfortunately, the scientific environment has become much more competitive. MD/PhDs may never develop the clinical skills and confidence to manage patients and lose the respect of clinicians. On the other hand, if the MD/PhDs pursue a basic sciences career they find themselves in a difficult position to compete for grants with PhDs who are not burdened or distracted by clinical responsibilities.

Furthermore, many bright and talented young physician scientists are unable to obtain grants or permanent academic or research positions.

In October 27, 2016 a special issue of Nature was devoted to "The plight of young scientists". Data show that despite doubling of the number of young people completing doctorate programs, there has been no growth in academic jobs. Furthermore, the rate for successfully obtaining research grants has declined below 20%. In contrast to 30 years ago, older scientists who better understand the system, are much more successful in obtaining grants than young scientists. The average age at which PhD scientists earn their first major grant is now around 42 years, much older than in the past.

In my view, supported by the special Nature issue, the major challenge for young researchers is the time it takes to apply for and administer grants as a result of which they have little or no time to actually plan and carry out experiments, analyze the data, and submit the findings into a high-impact journal. Furthermore, funding of clinical research increasingly relies on industry-driven trials, rather than investigator-initiated research [8]. This growing stress is compounded by the highly prevalent and ill-founded "publish or perish" philosophy that is dominating most academic faculty and promotion committees. To make the situation for junior researchers even more challenging is the growing emphasis on clinical productivity with "work RVU" as the new bench mark for faculty promotions. These increasing demands on clinical efficiency, coupled with stress associated with electronic medical records and increased administrative hassles has led to an exponential growth of physician burnout [9].

What advice would you give a young talented neurologist/ movement disorder expert?

Important ingredients of a happy and successful academic physician include:

- Family always comes first!
- Never recommend anything to your patients that you would not advise members of your own family
- Choose the best mentor in your or other academic/research environments
- In selecting an academic position be program rather than geography oriented
- Don't get discouraged by failures (e.g. rejected papers)
- Challenge your own decisions (and diagnoses) and others' dogmas
- Choose your battles and don't hold grudges if you lose
- Develop a unique skill (e.g. learn study design, statistics, regulatory requirements, scientific and grant-writing skills)
- As soon as the experiment is completed, analyze the data and submit for publication as efficiently as possible. Do not procrastinate.
- Choose a job you love, and you will never have to work a day in your life (Confucius).
- Ingredients to Happy and Successful Career: Curiosity, Ambition, Perseverance, Anticipation, Empathy, Integrity, and Luck! (CAPAEIL).

References

1. Jankovic J. Pathogenesis-targeted therapeutic strategies in Parkinson's disease. Mov Disord. 2019;34(1):41–4.
2. Jankovic J. Botulinum toxin: state of the art. Mov Disord. 2017;32(8):1131–8.

3. Jankovic J. Dopamine depleters in the treatment of hyperkinetic movement disorders. Expert Opin Pharmacother. 2016;17(18):2461–70.
4. Parsa-Parsi RW. The revised declaration of Geneva: a modern-day Physician's pledge. JAMA. 2017;318(20):1971–2.
5. Roberts BW, Walton K, Bogg T. Conscientiousness and health across the life course. Rev Gen Psychol. 2005;9:156–68.
6. Schor N. Pursuit and achievement of leadership: a view from the top. Ann Neurol. 2014;76(6):784–8.
7. Ropper A. How to determine if you have succeeded at Neurology residency. Ann Neurol. 2016;79:339–41.
8. Meador KJ. Decline of clinical research in academic medical centers. Neurology. 2015;85(13):1171–6.
9. Rotenstein LS, Torre M, Ramos MA, Rosales RC, Guille C, Sen S, Mata DA. Prevalence of burnout among physicians: a systematic review. JAMA. 2018;320(11):1131–50.

Chapter 20
JEON, Beomseok (BJ): Seoul/Republic of Korea

Bios Professor Beomseok Jeon is Medical Director of the Movement Disorder Center at Seoul National University Hospital. He is the past President of the Korean Movement Disorder Society, and served as the International Delegate of the Korean Neurological Association. He also served as the Director of Office of the Medical Policy and Communication, Seoul National University. Currently, he is Chair of MDS-AOS and President of the Asia-Oceanian Association of Neurology.

Prof. Jeon graduated from Seoul National University College of Medicine, and completed his neurology residency both at Seoul National University Hospital (1983–1987) and at the University of Minnesota (1987–1991), and then had movement disorder fellowship under Prof. Stanley Fahn at Columbia University (1991–1993). He also studied basic neurosciences under Prof. Robert Burke as H. Houston Merritt Fellow (1997–1998) at Columbia University.

B. Jeon (✉)
Seoul National University Hospital, Seoul, Republic of Korea
e-mail: brain@snu.ac.kr

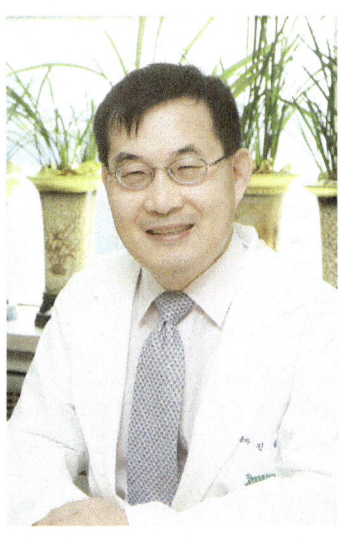

Reprinted with permission from Professor Beomseok Jeon

Why did you chose Neurology as a subspecialty?

Theodosius Dobzhansky, an evolutionary biologist, said "Nothing in biology makes sense except in the light of evolution."

When I look back and think whether I could have predicted or planned to be what I am now, I reflect I had very poor idea of what I will do and how I can achieve what I want to do. My life was just a series of adaptation to what was around me. Of course, I made some important choices, but choices were among what were available and around.

When I look back, it is amazing how I chose neurology when I had no systematized neuroscience education or great mentor during the medical school. In fact, I had no clear distinction between neurology, psychiatry and neurosurgery when I decided to enter into neurology. It was only several years and serendipitous events after that I wanted to pursue academic career in movement disorders. Convergent evolution is the process of evolving similar features in different species. A good example is the similar body shape of a shark and a dolphin, which are completely different species. They formed the similar body features because that body feature is the best underwater adaptation. Similarly, we may adapt. There may be lucky ones that can deliberately choose their path or are in the right place for their best growth. However, others may simply adapt to their surroundings and feel that they need to work against what they are in.

Who were your mentors? Do you remember life-changing encounters?

Before joining Seoul National University, I did my clinical training with Professor Stanley Fahn. I also received basic science training in order to best prepare myself in an academic center. My mentor in basic science was Professor Robert E. Burke, who was a meticulous and insightful thinker, and Professor Nikolai G. Kholodilov, who was an excellent molecular biologist. They were good teachers and I learned a lot. I worked on several basic science projects and wrote some papers. However, I had to give up because I realized that doing all by myself without getting much help was not fulfilling. Thus I concentrated on the clinical side: I had a busy clinical practice and did clinical research. This was much easier for me and very productive. In the water, I chose to have a fin rather than the leg.

Of course, my knowledge in basic science was not for nothing. It helped when I worked with my colleagues in genetics, and neuropathology. I was fortunate to work with very capable collaborators.

What are you most proud of with regards to your career achievements and development as a leader?

In 2005, I developed a movement disorder center that allows us to make best use of clinical data. It started with a good collaboration with our neurosurgeon Professor Sun Ha Paek. We together built the Movement Disorder Center that was more or less devoted to deep brain stimulation but also for monitoring patients. Timing was right to set up a big center: The Korean government made a decision to cover DBS. Thus the Hospital had a motive to move. With supporting staff and good facilities, it became much easier to collect clinical data systematically and analyze them at leisure. I worked hard, and very capable fellows joined in so it became a successful journey.

Philosophically spoken, I searched the resources around like filopodia and worked on them. I may have diverged out evolving into what I am because of a changing environment. The key word is adaptation. That is how any life form survives and prospers.

This slow process may apply to any sciences. "How do you start a revolution? Make changes as small as possible." Was it Werner Heisenberg, the great physicist, who said this? If you continue to make small but solid changes, you will end up making a revolution.

Chapter 21
TAN, Eng-King: Singapore/Singapore

Bios Professor Eng-King Tan is the Deputy Medical Director (Academic Affairs), Director, Research and a senior consultant with the Department of Neurology, National Neuroscience Institute (NNI). He is also a professor at the Duke-NUS Medical School and Lee Kong Chian School of Medicine. An influential figure in the field of research, Dr. Tan has authored more than 400 peer-reviewed papers and book chapters on clinical and neuroimaging studies, functional genomics and experimental therapeutics in Movement Disorders. He is presently an editor with European Journal of Neurology, Parkinsonism Related Disorders and Journal of Parkinson's disease. Dr. Tan has actively served in various committees in the International Movement Disorders Society (MDS) and the International Association Parkinsonism and Related Disorders (IAPRD) and is a founding member of the MDS Asian Oceanic Section. For his tremendous contribution to research in Movement Disorders, Dr. Tan has received numerous awards including 2016 Yoshikuni Mizuno Award, (MDS-Asian and Oceanian Section), 2018 David Marsden Award (MDS) and 2018 President's Science Award.

E.-K. Tan (✉)
National Neuroscience Institute, Duke NUS Medical School, Singapore, Singapore
e-mail: tan.eng.king@singhealth.com.sg

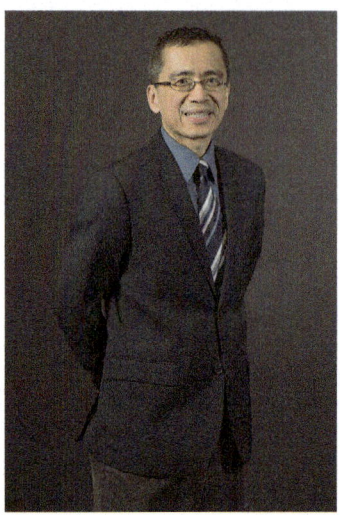

What were the key characteristics of your best mentor?

Extremely driven, passionate and yet level headed. These are the key factors that keep my mentors going and made them successful in their careers. Every one of my mentor has been excellent in their own individual ways and it would be unfair to rank them because in my mind, each one of them is the Best!

I was reminded that whatever contributions we make, it is only a tiny drop in the ocean. Essentially, the message is that no matter how successful we become, remember always to be humble and share your knowledge. Think this is the best advice from one of my mentors.

Is competition among a team healthy and constructive?

Competition is always healthy in any profession and in everyday life. However, if competition drives certain unethical, unprofessional and selfish behaviours, leading to disharmony, discord and unhealthy fights, then this usually will lead to more destructive behaviour and make any collaboration within the team untenable.

It is useful to have regular meetings among team members, be open and promote and encourage collaborative spirit and ensure team members are able to appreciate the win–win strategies being implemented.

This applies not just to a team but to any form of collaborations outside the team.

Have you ever taken on a job that you were unqualified for?

I have never been trained to take up higher job responsibilities involving handling finances and administration. So in many ways, I have always been unqualified to take on the various directorships and chairmanships of programmes and taskforces. However, many times we have to learn on the job and the unknown challenges I have taken on have benefitted me enormously as a person.

What are a few resources you would recommend to someone looking to gain insight into becoming a better leader?

One famous leader in my country reportedly said that you cannot become a good leader just by attending leadership courses. I agree partially with that view. However, I think attending leadership courses will enable one to appreciate the major challenges and potential solutions and ways to becoming a better leader. There are also many books on leadership, such as "The Leadership challenge" by James Kouzes and Barry Posner, and "Influence: The Psychology of persuasion" by Robert CIALDINI that are readily available as useful references.

The best resource is still the experience on the ground. We need to be able to take up the challenge when opportunity calls and gather advice from mentors how best to make use of the situation. I believe every one of us can become a leader, it is up to us to shape this in our own image.

Chapter 22
KISHORE, Asha: Kerala/India

Bios Asha Kishore is currently the Director of the Sree Chitra Tirunal Institute for Medical Sciences and Technology, an Institute of National Importance, under the Ministry of Science and Technology of the Government of India. She also holds the positions of Senior Grade Professor in the Department of Neurology and the Head of the Comprehensive Care Centre for Movement Disorders of the Institute. After her 2-year clinical research fellowship training in Movement Disorders with Professor Donald Calne, University of British Columbia, Vancouver, Canada, she returned to India in 1996, set up the first Comprehensive Care Centre for Movement Disorders in India at her institute and established the first MER- guided deep brain stimulation program in India. She has had the privilege to spend time in the Movement Disorder Programs led by Professors Mahlon Delong, USA, Alim Louis Benabid, Grenoble, Antony Lang, Toronto, Professor Kailash Bhatia, London and Marie Vidailet, Paris. Under the guidance and inspiration of Professor Mark Hallet and Dr. Sabine Meunier, INSERM, Paris, she has also set up a Motor physiology and Transcranial Magnetic Stimulation Lab for Movement Disorders in India. She is also one of the leading researchers working in the field of genetics of Parkinson's disease in collaboration with Manu Sharma, University of Tubingen. Asha had the privilege of training over 150 neurology residents, PhD students and post-doctoral fellows. She is also one of the founding members of the Movement Disorder Society of India and former executive committee member of MDS-AOS.

A. Kishore (✉)
Comprehensive Care Centre for Movement Disorders, Sree Chitra Tirunal Institute for medical Sciences and Technology, Thiruvananthapuram, Kerala, India
e-mail: asha@sctimst.ac.in; director@sctimst.ac.in

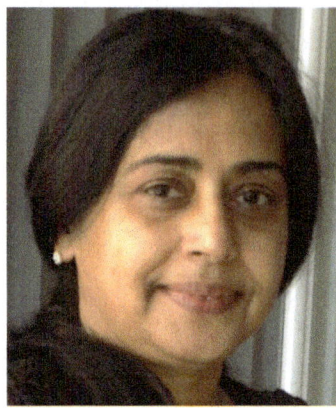

Reprinted with permission from Prof. Asha Kishore

How do you build team morale?

As the head of the Movement Disorders program and as the Director of a national institute with diverse mandates and faculties, I recognised that to achieve any goal, the first step is to build a good team and generate excitement among the members of the team and make them feel passionate about achieving our collective goal through the best performance of the team and its members. If the leader is energetic and dynamic, it enthuses the team. I make it a point to express confidence in the team and their abilities which helps to boost the team of the morale. I am genuine and honest in all interactions with the team which is important to earn their trust. Opinions and ideas need to be invited to create a sense of ownership and incorporated when they are good and acknowledged too. Problem solving strategy, clear role assignments, setting time lines, decision making rules etc. must be in place to build confidence in team members. Besides tact and diplomacy, it helps to have a good sense of humour and to be able to laugh at oneself when one is leading a time through tough times. It is important to be optimistic about a positive outcome but at the same time let them know that failure should be treated a great learning experience to ensure future success. It helps to share stories of personal success and failures with the team and how one learns to handle both. I find that a team tries harder to avert failure if the leader accepts that the final responsibility for failure rests with the leader. However, the leader must be available to help them fix problems and overcome hurdles. If things don't work out and results are not forthcoming, new ways have to be identified and a leader should be able to innovate and change strategies. Team members should feel valued. Their achievements have to be openly recognized and appreciated. This is yet another morale booster. As a leader I strive to create or provide opportunities for the members to get exposure and opportunities for them to be recognized for their work and get noticed in academic circles. It was important as a leader to ensure that the success of teamwork enhances the career prospects of the members. Young members may need mentoring and guidance and links with external agencies or teams that the leader may have already established. It is necessary to be empathetic and supportive when members have personal difficulties even if outside of the work place. While encouraging the young members to develop their own strengths and settle their own issues, their morale goes up if the leader can establish good rapport with the members and show gestures with a personal touch every now and then and be attentive to the well-being and personal growth of the members. Social activities must be encouraged so that the members get to know each other at different levels and in different environments as team unity is paramount. I have been greatly impressed by Dr. Donald Cane, former Director of the Neurodegenerative Disorders centre at the University of Vancouver, a brilliant clinician and researcher with razor sharp intellect under whom I trained. He and his wife Susan treated the research team like their own family, inspired them, cared for them and helped them in all ways they could. Prof. Cane brought out the best in his people and ensured success in all the major challenges he took up.

How do you lead through change?

One of the greatest challenges to leadership that I have experienced as head of an Institution is that my leadership counts when I am able to make major change that was long pending and much needed but avoided for fear of resistance. There is always resistance to change and it can be hostile and threaten leadership. So as a leader I had to prepare myself to take the heat and survive the difficulties. I had to have a clear vision and understanding of the need to change, weigh the risks versus benefits, analyze the existing situation and prevailing sentiments, understand the issues that were likely to be raised, the stakes and the pace of change appropriate for the people in the Institution.

It is important to convey that changes are not for the personal gain or advancement but for common good, if not the immediate or short term but in the foreseeable long term. The future and opportunities and advantages have to be clearly enunciated to the people in multiple ways. People need to be convinced that the stakes are worth the difficulties they may suffer. The information provided has to be clear and convincing and non threatening. It is wise to test the waters and get a sense of the thinking of the key people who are likely to oppose. Changing status quo always generates unrest, resentment and anxiety. If the leader appreciates the sacrifices or compromises that people are making, they are likely to be less resentful of the change. It is important to remember that the opposition is generally because it gives a sense of disruption of their stability and uncertainty about the future. This is directed at the leader as he is in the position to make the decision to change. It is vital not to take it personally as it may cloud one's judgement. Once an action is taken, it is necessary to assess the action and the reaction. It is necessary to listen to view points of others and accept constructive criticism rather than remain adamant about the logic of one's own argument. Even if the leader strives to take everyone along, it is not always possible. I have found it necessary to deal firmly with those who are disruptive and create mayhem at the place of work in order to resist change. Dissent may be allowed but the leader should have control. Once the heat settles, draw up time lines, implement the first phase of change and create a small momentum of activity. Too much too soon is bound to fail. Spreading the implementation over a longer period of time will give those affected a chance to assess the new versus old. One can always reassess one's action after seeing people's reaction and take ongoing corrective action, if needed. If people get a glimpse of the future through early results, they are less likely to fixate on their difficulties and will participate in the process of change.

What was the biggest risk you have taken in your role as a leader?

Resisting political and other external interference while implementing financial regulations necessary for the progress of the institution, restructuring academic departments, applying objective measure to assess merit and productivity for promotions and instituting promotion criteria to enhance productivity and scientific contribution by the faculty.

How do you measure success for you as a leader?

I feel that I have succeeded when the team/institution is able deliver high quality work exceeding expectations. There is a sense of personal success when with or without me around, the team that I nurture can generate new ideas, plan strategies, fix problems, navigate through turbulent situations and deliver results with a sense of autonomy, responsibility and accountability. If I see that excitement and passion have become a way of life at the work place, that the teams will not falter in absence, will care for each other's welfare and the future of the institution, I feel that my job can then be considered successful.

How can a leader fail?

Leaders fail when they cannot envision, execute change, are not willing to take risks or handle dissent. If they become self-absorbed and promote only themselves, demonstrate hunger for power and control and do not share credit or acknowledge others, colleagues avoid them. If a leader has no integrity, honesty, passion or enthusiasm and is not capable of taking responsibility, dealing with failure and disappointment, the team will lose faith and confidence very quickly.

Chapter 23
KLEIN, Christine: Luebeck/Germany

Bios Dr. Christine Klein is a Professor of Neurology and Neurogenetics. She studied medicine in Hamburg, Heidelberg, Luebeck, London, and Oxford. She moved to Boston from 1997 to 1999 for a fellowship in Molecular Neurogenetics with Dr. X. O. Breakefield and completed her neurology training at Luebeck University in 2004, followed by a series of summer sabbaticals in movement disorders with Dr. A. E. Lang in Toronto, Canada in 2004–2015. She was appointed Lichtenberg Professor at the Department of Neurology of Luebeck University in 2005, where her research has focused on the clinical and molecular genetics of movement disorders and its functional consequences. In 2009, Dr. Klein been appointed Schilling Professor of Clinical and Molecular Neurogenetics at the University of Luebeck and became Director of the newly founded Institute of Neurogenetics in 2013.

Dr. Klein has published over 400 scientific papers and has an h-factor of 84. She is an Associate Editor of 'Annals of Neurology' and of 'Movement Disorders', served as chair of the Congress Scientific Program Committee of the 2016/2017 Annual Congresses of the International Parkinson and Movement Disorder Society, and will become President of the German Neurological Society (>9500 members) in 2019. Nine of her former doctoral students or mentees have been promoted to the level of assistant, associate or even full professor.

C. Klein (✉)
Neurogenetics and Neurology, Institute of Neurogenetics, University Hospital of Schleswig-Holstein, University of Luebeck, Luebeck, Germany
e-mail: christine.klein@neuro.uni-luebeck.de; http://neurogenetics-luebeck.de

© Springer Nature Switzerland AG 2019
S. A. Schneider, C. Comella (eds.), *Leadership in Movement Disorders*,
https://doi.org/10.1007/978-3-030-12967-5_23

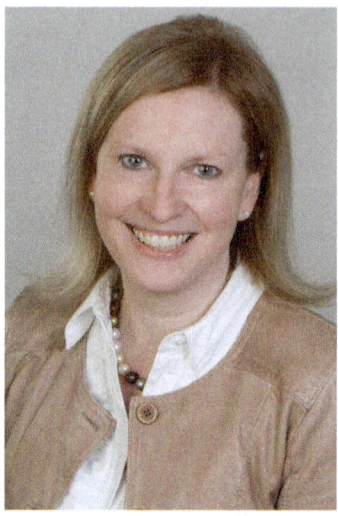

Reprinted with permission from Professor Christine Klein

What is your leadership philosophy?

Leadership is all about building a strong team of colleagues, coworkers and students who all work towards the same goal. In the case of our clinical and research focus at the Institute of Neurogenetics, University of Luebeck, Germany, we aim to diagnose and treat patients with (hereditary) movement disorders in the best possible way and to understand the underlying disease causes in order to further improve therapeutic options. Naturally, our team includes members with very different expertise ranging from clinical to basic science and with variable levels of education and career goals. Thus, leadership needs to be both 'broad' and 'deep', integrating across different needs, expectations, and opportunities. A good leader needs to be fair, however, at the same time, it can be unfair to treat everyone the same way. Therefore, a leader needs to be able to strike a good balance between treating all members of the group equally to a certain extent, while also tailoring to individual requirements and talents. Very importantly, this philosophy needs to be obvious and transparent. Leadership ideally should facilitate career development and good working conditions as much as possible, while reinforcing rules whenever necessary in a predictable fashion. One final 'leadership pearl' I would like to share is: Always try to recruit the best people to your team ('A hires A') and avoid a 'B hires C' situation. In many cases adding brilliant people to your team will mean that they are better in certain areas than you are—seize the opportunity to learn from them, as you and your team will both grow and benefit.

Where do the great ideas come from in your organization?

Great ideas come from everyone and are contributed at every level. For example, a technician may propose an excellent way of simplifying an assay saving both time and money, a clinician scientist can make an astute observation that may lead to a previously unrecognized diagnostic or treatment option or a basic scientist can uncover a novel disease mechanism paving the way towards new therapeutic approaches. It can sometimes be challenging to tell apart a great idea from a perhaps not so great one and to allocate time and resources accordingly when it comes to pursuing such ideas. Excellent ideas are often sparked by deep knowledge of the field; thus, carefully and regularly reading scientific literature and attending meetings for scientific exchange are strongly encouraged. Finally, great ideas are best born in an environment where any idea can be voiced and discussed in an open and respectful manner and where one can be sure that the 'IP' related to this idea will be recognized by everyone.

How do you set an example to your team members?

I am trying to be available to my team members as much as possible which includes regular group but also one-on-one meetings. Some decisions are less popular than others; I always try to be predictable, reliable and consistent. One of my goals it to clearly define responsibilities, as well as benefits, which I expect from the group leaders at the Institute in a similar way. I pay as much careful attention to detail as possible, as this is an indispensable prerequisite for producing high-quality data, papers, theses etc. I try to keep learning as much as possible and encourage my team members to do the same. I am working hard and try to contribute personally whenever needed. It is important to find the right balance between delegating certain tasks—which of course helps economizing workflows—and performing certain jobs oneself. After all, no one is 'too important' or could not use a short break to, for example, empty the dish washer once in a while…

Was there a time when you had to make a decision without all the relevant facts?

With a growing team of ~80 colleagues and co-workers at the Institute of Neurogenetics and increasingly complex, interdisciplinary, and international research projects, having to make a decision without all of the relevant facts seems to be a considerable risk and difficult to avoid. In fact, at times, it can be difficult to even know where to gather all of the relevant facts or what all of the relevant facts may be. For this very reason, important decisions have to be taking with great care and are often based on team consensus. As it is probably unavoidable that 'wrong' decisions are made at times, it is helpful to closely monitor the consequences of decisions and to retract or modify a decision if necessary. After all, nobody is perfect but success tends to be based on the sum of right decisions.

Chapter 24
KONING-TIJSSEN, Marina AJ de: Groningen/The Netherlands

Bios Prof. Marina A. J. de Koning-Tijssen was trained as a neurologist at the Leiden University Medical Centre, The Netherlands. She defended her thesis 'Hyperekplexia' in 1997. As a research fellow she worked with Prof. David S. Zee, Johns Hopkins University, Baltimore, USA and with Prof. Peter Brown at the Institute of Neurology, Queen Square, London, UK. In the period 1999-2012, she worked as a neurologist and principal investigator in the Academic Medical Center in Amsterdam. Since 2012 she is head of the Movement Disorder section, department of Neurology at the University Medical Center Groningen and chair of the Groningen Expertise Center for rare Movement Disorders, part of an European Network. Nationally, she chaired the Dutch Movement Society and is head of DystoniaNet. Internationally, she chaired the clinical line of the European COST platform Dystonia. Currently, she is part of the Rare disorders committee of the European Academy of Neurology, member of several MDS task forces and committees, and secretary of the European Section of the MDS.

Her research 'Hyperkinetic movement disorders' ranges from basic research to patient care with a focus on phenotyping, genetic and functional (neurophysiology and imaging) studies. Clinical studies focus on the motor and non-motor aspects of movement disorders.

M. A. J. de Koning-Tijssen (✉)
Movement Disorders, Department of Neurology, University Medical Center Groningen, University of Groningen, Groningen, The Netherlands
e-mail: M.A.J.de.Koning-Tijssen@umcg.nl; http://movementdisordersgroningen.com

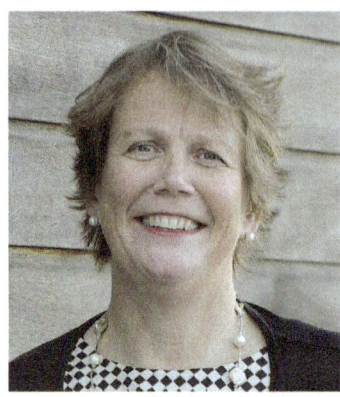

Reprinted with permission from Prof. Marina A. J. de Koning-Tijssen

How did you become a leader in your field?

The main reason I became a leader in my field is that I really enjoy my work. I love the combination of clinical work, research and education in movement disorders. Over time, I learned from my teachers. In Leiden, Prof. Gert van Dijk taught me the fundamental basics of research and thereby gave me confidence to do my own research. During my fellowships with David Zee at the John Hopkins and with Peter Brown and Andrew Lees at Queen Square I learned from top level (eye) movement disorder specialists. Being taught neurology and movement disorders by international recognised experts was the foundation to build an international network, and to become a good movement disorder specialist. Equally important to me is the fact that I enjoy (family) life.

These skills enabled me to start as a neurologist in Amsterdam. A major step forward to further extend my own research group was a prestigious Dutch VIDI-grant (2004) for my project "Myoclonic dystonia: borderland between neurology and psychiatry". In 2012, I became a professor in Movement Disorders in Groningen, supported by a fantastic group of people. By joining the European COST initiative, MDS committees, and becoming secretary of the MDS-ES I experienced the pleasure of leadership, collaboration, and to make friends.

What do you like about managing and leading people?

I enjoy inspiring young people in the field of movement disorders and guide them both clinically as well as in their research endeavours. My style is to give personal attention and support, and to create a safe and supportive atmosphere so my junior colleagues develop their own skills. I feel it is important to have a clear view on people's potentials and encourage them to play to their strengths. In addition, I enjoy bringing together a group of people and constructing a close team with a shared sense of purpose, while also having a good time together.

What is one mistake you witness leaders making more frequently than others?

I believe the main challenge of being a leader is to be aware of your own limitations. It is essential to have colleagues that feel free to give honest and direct feedback, to improve your leadership skills. Over the years, I have noticed that people in high ranking positions are not necessarily top notch when it comes to people management. I think it is a mistake to let your own drive and ambition stand in the way of being a great leader to serve others.

Do you have advise addressed to young females in their early career ?

I would like to encourage them to be as ambitious as they want to be. Be yourself, take on board the femininity you have and do not strive to be like a man. If you decide you want a family then take your time for that: allow yourself the time and enjoy it. After you have settled in, it will be easier to go forwards again. Please make sure you arrange things as best as you can to make life a little easier. In my opinion, this means investing in care and support for your household, you can't do everything yourself. To me it has always felt like a privilege to be a good movement disorder specialist and to have a family.

Chapter 25
LANG, Anthony: Ontario/Canada

Bios Dr. Anthony Lang trained in Internal Medicine and Neurology at the University of Toronto, followed by a postgraduate training in Movement Disorders in London, England under the late Professor David Marsden. He initiated and continues to direct the Toronto Western Hospital Movement Disorders Clinic which is now one of the best know programs in movement disorders in the world with 9 full-time faculty members (each with international renown), 7 nurses, up to 10 fellows and a staff of over 30. He holds the Jack Clark Chair for Parkinson's Disease Research at the University of Toronto and Lily Safra Chair in Movement Disorders at the Toronto Western Hospital.

Dr. Lang served on the International Parkinson and Movement Disorder Society (MDS) Executive Committee in several capacities over the years: as Treasurer from 1988 to 1992, Secretary from 1996 to 1998 and then President from 2007 to 2009. He was Co-editor-in-Chief of the Society's journal *Movement Disorders* between 1996 and 2003. In 2011, he was listed as the most highly cited investigator in the field of Parkinson's disease for the decade 2001–2009.

A. E. Lang (✉)
Edmond J Safra Program in Parkinson's Disease, Morton and Gloria Shulman Movement Disorders Clinic, Toronto Western Hospital, Toronto, ON, Canada
e-mail: lang@uhnresearch.ca

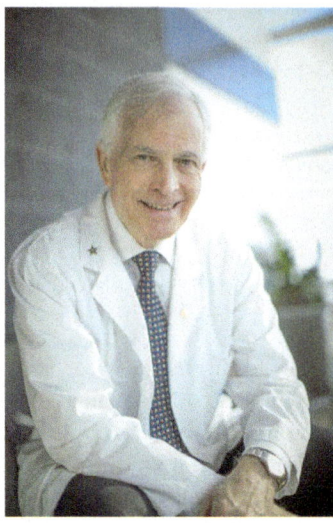

Reprinted with permission from Dr. Anthony Lang

In your mind, what are the main clues towards a successful career?

From my perspective, the most important factors that influence a successful career include perseverance, hard work, good collaborating skills and team spirit, organizational skills and especially love for what you do. In addition, it's extremely important to have strong interpersonal skills and emotional intelligence.

What is your greatest strength as a leader?

I believe that my strength as a leader relates to the fact that I am open to everyone's ideas and supportive of others but able to make the final, sometimes difficult, decisions.

What do you find are the most difficult leadership decisions to make?

I find that the most challenging aspects of leadership relate to difficult personalities and egos. Probably like everyone, I find confrontation extremely difficult to deal with and this can sometimes challenge leadership decisions considerably. Related to this, reprimanding or punishing an employee/research team member for major misbehavior and eventually dismissing them are very difficult decisions and also very challenging given selected working environments.

What do you like to ask other leaders when you get the chance?

When meeting other leaders I will often ask similar questions to those listed above. I am always struck by how prolific and successful some colleagues are and always interested in what has made this possible, particularly in people who are extremely busy and highly productive.

Chapter 26
LITVAN, Irene: California/USA

Bios Dr. Litvan is the Tasch Endowed Chair of Parkinson Disease Research at the University of California San Diego (UCSD), Professor of Neurosciences and Director of the UCSD Parkinson and Other Movement Disorder Center of Excellence. She earned her MD degree in Uruguay and completed Neurological and Neuropsychological training in Barcelona, Spain and a Neurology Residency at Georgetown, DC. She spent nine years at the National Institutes of Health, was visiting fellow at the Experimental Therapeutic Branch and Senior Staff fellow at the Neuroepidemiology Branch, and Human Motor Control Section. She was elected fellow at the American Neurological Association and is an American Academy of Neurology (AAN) fellow. Currently, she is the Chair of the International Parkinson Movement Disorder Society (IP-MDS) Continuous Medical Education Committee, World Federation of Neurology Dementia section secretary, and AAN Movement Disorder Section past Chair. She is member of multiple layman advisory boards and scientific committees. Dr. Litvan has led multiple multicenter studies and international Task Forces to develop clinical and neuropathologic diagnostic criteria for all parkinsonian and non-Alzheimer dementia neurodegenerative disorders. Dr. Litvan published more than 300 peer-reviewed articles and is senior coeditor of 4 books. She was co-Editor of Moving Along and is Chief Editor of *Frontiers in Neurology*. She built an Interdisciplinary Movement Disorder Center at the University of Louisville and another at UCSD. Both were designated National Parkinson Foundation Center of Excellence. The UCSD Center was also designated Research Center of Excellence in Lewy Body Dementia and CurePSP Center of Care. She has mentored several US and international fellows who have become leaders in their own countries.

I. Litvan (✉)
Department of Neurosciences, UC San Diego School of Medicine, La Jolla, CA, USA

Parkinson and Other Movement Disorders Center, Altman Clinical Translational Research Institute, La Jolla, CA, USA
e-mail: ilitvan@ucsd.edu

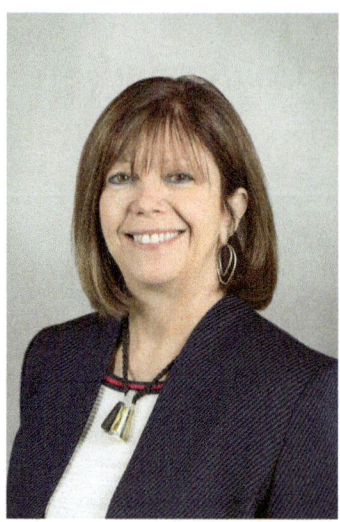

Reprinted with permission from Dr. Irene Litvan

What is the most significant change that you brought to an organization? When I was elected as Chair of American Academy of Neurology Movement (AAN) Disorder Section, the prior section Chairs told us that the AAN leadership was not interested in collaborating with the International Parkinson Movement Disorder Society (IP-MDS). To overcome this problem, I separately met the leaders of both organizations and explained that this collaboration could be a win-win situation and this was a timely moment to collaborate. Through the AAN, residents could be exposed early to movement disorders specialists increasing the number of specialists. On the other hand, the AAN could improve their educational courses in movement disorders and the care to our patients by accessing to our educational courses and our expertise. To develop AAN trust, it was timely that the IP-MDS President (Chris Goetz) and PAS elect chair (Cindy Comella) were well known AAN leaders. Persistence did the rest. Timeliness, persistence, and clear goals allowed starting a collaboration that is improving awareness and education on movement disorders.

What sort of leader would your team say that you are?

My team says that my approach is democratic and I inspire them to achieve a shared mission, goals and tasks that assure the benefit of everyone. I strive to operate as an orchestra conductor and I encourage the group's participation and co-operation. They appreciate that I rarely give up.

What kind of criticism you most get?

The most common ones are that I work too much or I trust people too much. Some millennials' feel that I may demand more than what they want to commit.

How do you get others to accept your ideas?

I believe that the example given above is a typical and practical method. I clearly present my ideas and goals to those involved, taking their interests into consideration. I strive to show how individuals or group can benefit from cooperating in accomplishing the goals. This process occasionally is slow, thus requiring patience and perseverance. I have multiple examples of demonstrated perseverance. When a political dictatorship in Uruguay closed the University, I continued my medical studies in Buenos Aires, Argentina. Fortunately, after a few months in Argentina, the University reopened in Uruguay and I returned to complete my studies. When I became a physician, I decided not to stay in a repressive society. I was told by the Spanish embassy that Spain needed doctors. I left the dictatorship in Uruguay, and moved to Spain. However, upon arriving in Spain, I discovered a different situation. The Spanish government had ruled that foreigners were not allowed to compete for residency positions because they had positions for the thousands of Spanish and South Americans competing for residencies. My passion for medicine motivated me to become a volunteer in three hospitals in Barcelona. Unexpectedly, I came across an opening for a residency position that did not reject foreigners, and I applied to it. I ranked first in the competition, but then the hospital refused to accept me, based on government's rules. Subsequently, I formally challenged the hospital's policy, and was given an opportunity to take a new oral exam. After passing first the oral exam, the hospital accepted me, and I was assigned a position in family medicine. However, because Neurology was my passion, I resigned and volunteered in the Neurology department. I waited many months for an opportunity to compete and got the first position. After becoming a neurologist, I focused my career on clinical research, and I relocated to the USA. Adjusting to different cultures and repeating my neurology residency in the USA required perseverance. I'm extremely thankful that I was able to adjust to all my challenges in the various transitions. The passion for what I do energizes me, and propels me to overcome the many challenges that are in front of me. I believe people should never give up, and should be willing to struggle on the path to reaching their goals.

How do you deal with failure?

I learned from my oldest brother that each failure is an opportunity to succeed. I try to understand what led to the failure, work on how to overcome it and wait for new opportunities. Perseverance is extremely important to overcome set-backs.

How can a leader fail?

Leaders fail when they are autocratic, believe their mission is to pursue their own goals, don't communicate with their team, promise what they cannot deliver, don't inspire and don't allow the team members to flourish.

Chapter 27
MERELLO, Marcelo: Buenos Aires/Argentina

Bios Born in Argentina in 1961, Marcelo J. Merello graduated from Buenos Aires University School of Medicine in 1987, where later on he obtained his Ph.D. degree. In Buenos Aires, he completed first, an Internal Medicine residency program at CEMIC and then one in Neurology at FLENI. He was also Research Fellow in Neurology at the National Hospital for Neurology and Neurosurgery, Queen Square and Research Registrar in Neurology at Middlesex Hospital, both in London. Currently, he is Head of the Movement Disorders Section at the Raul Carrea Institute for Neurological Research (FLENI) in Buenos Aires and Director of Neuroscience at the same institution. He is Chair of Post Graduate Neurology at the University of Buenos Aires and Professor of Neurology at the Pontificia Universidad Catolica Argentina (UCA). He also works as Clinical Researcher for National Scientific and Technical Research Council (CONICET) in Argentina.

He has co-authored over 250 papers in leading peer review journals in the field of Movement Disorders and more than 20 book chapters. He has written/co-edited six books, and been member of the editorial board of the Movement Disorders Journal. Member of the IEC of the IP-MDS, founding editor of the IPMDS website, he is currently co-editor in chief of the journal: Movement Disorders Clinical Practice.

M. Merello (✉)
Department of Neuroscience (FLENI), Clinical Researcher for National Scientific and Technical Research Council (CONICET), Buenos Aires, Argentina
e-mail: mmerello@fleni.org.ar

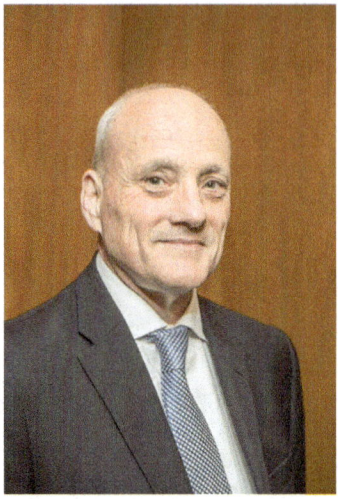

Reprinted with permission from Professor Marcelo J. Merello

Do you remember a life-changing academic experience or clinical encounter?

All my encounters and academic experiences have been enriching. Even negative role models have been important to realize who one does want to become, or what one does not want to do. There is no doubt in my mind that I chose to become a Neurologist as a result of a thrilling experience during my third year of medical school, when I met Professor Ramon Leiguarda, and was impressed by his outstanding clinical skills and overall charisma. Many years later, after finishing my neurology training, I went to study movement disorders at UCL College London and at the National Hospital at Queen Square. The reader is probably not aware that at that time internet and email did not exist, nor did the International Movement Disorders Congress. So, it´s not easy to explain the impact that putting a face to the names I had read about, and whose work I had admired for years, had on me at this time. My mentor, Andrew Lees was there. I may write a book on Andrew someday, using the same words that he used just few weeks ago when referring to Gerald Stern *"I owe him almost everything in my career"*. After meeting him, I knew who the role model to follow was going to be for me.

Not much later, as I sat in the corner of a small office full of secretaries, one of them called out to Dr. Quinn, as it happens I had just published my one and only paper in a relatively small new journal called Movement Disorders, and my first reference in it had been from a paper by Niall Quinn. Later during the same week I came across a "Journal Editor" for first time in my life, when I saw David Marsden walking alone down a long corridor smoking a cigarette seemingly escaping from the crowd. I cannot forget to mention Gerald Stern, who played squash with me once a week, and despite a significant age difference in my favor, beat me every time. Gerald was a wise person, I remember the first time I had to give a lecture in English at one of the earlier MDS meetings, he spent over an hour helping me with it. "Don't read the slides" he said, "People know how to read". These individuals I had read about for years turned out to be real, approachable people, helpful and eager to guide me. One message I would pass on to young physicians is, never hesitate to contact professors, no matter how important or distinguished they are in the field, it has been my experience that they will always open their door to you.

Are there specific challenges for those from under-represented areas ?

As a Latin-American physician, I believe a great gap still exists between basic research activities and clinical practice. Perhaps my experience cannot be universally generalized, but for physicians from the region or areas with similar problems, I believe this is a commonly shared belief. Even though three Nobel prices have been awarded to Argentinean scientists, two for medicine and one for chemistry and the University is well recognized worldwide, academic and research activities have no real impact on hospital positions or level of remuneration for local practicing physicians, which in turn has had a negative effect on young people striving to strike a career balance between clinical practice, research and teaching.

The second issue that young doctors have to face in under-represented areas is scientific isolation, despite the fact that most large meeting and congress venues rotate around the world. Smaller educational meetings, where the opportunity to interact closely with the most relevant leaders in the field occurs, including grand rounds, small institution symposia and collaborative work opportunities generally take place in North America and Europe. Although this limitation may have substantially improved today thanks to the Internet, it remains difficult for young doctors in the southern hemisphere to establish successful international academic careers. The experience and advice I share here should therefore be read in this context.

Have you ever considered leaving the career path you were on in order to do something else (completely different or somewhat related)? What influenced you to stay and keep going?

As I get older and I have more interests outside medicine. I often consider whether the time has come to quit my profession. However, the fellows that make up my work group, my students and my patients renew my interest in Movement Disorders day after day. So, my advice is to avoid isolation, to work in teams and try to put together a dedicated group of people. This I believe is the key to a productive and overall enjoyable career. I have never learnt as much about movement disorders as I have since I was appointed Editor for Movement Disorders Clinical Practice, not only from my Co-editor Kailash Bhatia, but also from the authors and reviewers contributing to the publication. Becoming a reviewer is an interesting way to renew one's passion for this fascinating field.

What are the challenges for a young scientist/academic/ clinician today compared to the past and how to tackle them?

The Index Medicus and letters posted through the regular mail service have been replaced by PubMed and emails. The advantages of these modern tools, now available to everyone, require no explanation. However, they have reduced the time for reflection and increased anxiety levels in young doctors. Anxiety over the need to publish rapidly, to be cited in papers by others, and be recognized. Young doctors and fellows need to understand that a career takes time. If you are not invited to deliver a talk at a meeting, don't be frustrated. Just stand in front of your poster, be proud of it and treat every visitor occasionally passing by it as your qualified audience. I have always seen the most productive, clever people and journal editors silently walking around the posters. Don't be frustrated if your papers are not accepted, start with small pieces in local journals and keep trying.

Read at least once in your career, the outstanding article by Richard Asher published in the Lancet in 1949 on the Seven Sins of Medicine. I would like to point out one of the sins described in the paper in particular, "Spanophilia" or the love of rarities. Remember that overall, we are clinicians and that even though sometimes they may present in an unusual manner, the majority of conditions affecting patients are common ones many of which are curable. Do not be misled or blinded by rarities. Exome sequencing is great, but don't forget to use your hammer when examining patients, to practice good clinical observation, to talk to your patients and even more importantly, to listen to them, something we often forget to do.

Chapter 28
OBESO, Jose: Madrid/Spain

Bios Jose A. Obeso trained in Neurology in San Sebastian. He spent 2 years in the Institute of Psychiatry training in movement disorders with C. David Marsden. He developed most of his professional career in the University of Navarra in Pamplona Spain; he is now director of the Neuroscience centre (CINAC) in HM Puerta del Sur Hospital in south of Madrid (Mostoles) and full professor of Neurology in CEU-San Pablo University in Madrid. He is honorary member and Invited Professor of several organizations and institutions such as the Colombian Neurological Association, Bolivian Neurological Association and Universidad de La Habana. He is current Editor in Chief of the Movement Disorders Journal.

He has pioneered (along with other researchers like Tom Chase and Fabriccio Stochi) the development of the concept of "Continuous dopaminergic stimulation" for Parkinson's disease, defined mechanisms associated with myoclonus, tics and dystonia and played a significant role in the revitalization of surgical treatments for Parkinson's disease in the 1990s. He trained more than 50 fellows and PhD students in the fields of neurology and movement disorders and published more than 350 peer-reviewed papers.

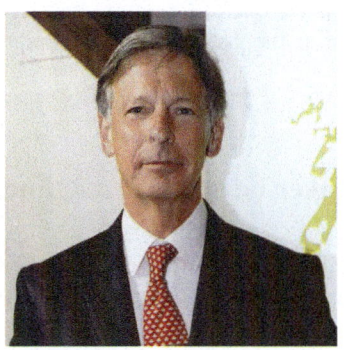

Reprinted with permission from Prof. Jose A. Obeso

J. A. Obeso (✉)
Centro Integral de Neurociencias AC (CINAC), Hospital Universitario HM Puerta del Sur, Madrid, Spain

© Springer Nature Switzerland AG 2019
S. A. Schneider, C. Comella (eds.), *Leadership in Movement Disorders*,
https://doi.org/10.1007/978-3-030-12967-5_28

What is your leadership philosophy?

First of all, work hard and don't ask junior and assistant colleagues what I am not prepared to do. Second, to listen to the team and try to take up suggestions and criticisms. Third, realize and put in practice that in current medicine, the Professor (the leader) is not the one who is more expert and knowledgeable on everything.

What advice would you give a young talented neurologist/movement disorder expert?

First of all, to make sure he/she learns very well the fundamental principles of neurology/movement disorders. It is essential not to lose ground with symptoms and signs, recognize them appropriately and put them into the right perspective. Secondly, set to resolve an issue. Ask yourself, what do I want to understand and move forward? And fight hard to accomplish it.

What is one mistake you witness leaders making more frequently than others?

I think the sub-speciality of movement disorders is privilege in that leaders, historically, have been away of super-ego behavior/attitude, and have enjoyed by and a large quite good sensitivity and humor. In any case, if I have to say a frequent nowadays "mistake" that I see is the one of forgetting the critical importance of clinical skills, phenomenology and pathophysiology. This is potentially dangerous for our area.

Should a decision maker be right all the time?

Of course not! This is out of question. The real point is how the leader reacts to error making. How long it takes to realize/recognize it and what is the next action.

Has there been a time as a leader when you changed an opinion after acquiring new facts and data. How did you communicate this to your team?

Keep, I think (you would need to ask people who has worked with me or are now working with me!!), a rather open approach to decision making. I like to make the team to feel and believe every opinion counts. Of course, at the end of the day, the leader/responsible person has to take decisions. The very final step of decision making can't be an entirely democratic process in academic medicine (and in many other aspects of life), but most of the process is open to questioning, opinions, discussion, etc.

Chapter 29
OKUBADEJO, Njideka Ulunma: Lagos State/Nigeria

Bios Njideka U. Okubadejo is a Professor of Neurology and Consultant Neurologist specializing in Movement Disorders at the College of Medicine, University of Lagos, Nigeria. She trained at the National Postgraduate Medical College of Nigeria (1992–1998), with additional observership at Howard University, Washington DC (1997/98), and a Visiting Clinical Fellowship in Movement Disorders sponsored by the Mayo Clinic, Rochester, Minnesota in 2004/2005. She is the first female neurologist and first female tenured Professor of Neurology in Nigeria. She is an American Academy of Neurology Donald M. Palatucci Advocacy Leadership Forum (PALF) member (class of 2009), and the 2015 awardee of the Society of Neuroscientists in Africa (SONA)/International Brain Research Organization (IBRO) Women in Neuroscience Award (West African Subregion). Prof. Okubadejo has worked extensively with the International Parkinson and Movement Disorders Society (MDS) to promote movement disorders education and quality of care in Africa, and serves as faculty and course director for trainings across sub Saharan Africa. She is the current chair of the MDS Africa Section Steering Committee, chair of the Neurology Subspecialty of the Faculty of Internal Medicine, National Postgraduate College of Nigeria, and member of the Scientific Committee, African Academy of Neurology. Her main research interest is in Movement Disorders in Africa (particularly genetics and epidemiology).

N. U. Okubadejo (✉)
Neurology Unit, Department of Medicine, Faculty of Clinical Sciences, College of Medicine, Lagos University Teaching Hospital, University of Lagos, Idi Araba, Lagos, Nigeria
e-mail: nokubadejo@unilag.edu.ng

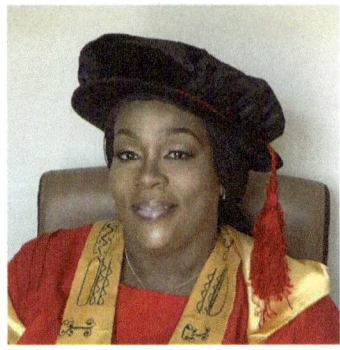

Reprinted with permission from Prof. Njideka U. Okubadejo

What are you most proud of with regards to your career achievements and development as a leader?

Probably the most important achievement for me has been the opportunity to inspire a love for neurology and mentor young neurologists in my country, and more recently across Africa. As I have grown in the course of my career, the importance of sustaining this passion for movement disorders has become clear, with the ultimate goal of building a generation of neurologists with not just knowledge and skills, but with a palpable passion to improve the quality of care and outcomes of each patient that they have the privilege to care for. At the time I delved (or dived more like) into neurology as a resident doctor in 1994, no female had dared to specialize in the field, in a country in which a formal residency training program had been in place for at least three decades prior. I ventured, and ultimately demonstrated that it was indeed doable. I am gladdened by the fact that subsequently, and over the course of my career since becoming my country's first female neurologist, at least 10 others have followed suit. My foray into Movement Disorders was no different—prior to expressing an interest in gaining expertise in Parkinson disease and other movement disorders, no one had been specifically trained in the subspecialty in my country. I am proud that following my training, and opportunities to share the knowledge gained and expose others to learning opportunities through international networks such as the International Parkinson and Movement Disorder Society, the number of neurologists with a special interest in movement disorders in my country and across the sub Saharan Africa region has grown.

How can a leader fail?

By failing to do that which is required—failing to lead. Leading by example is perhaps the surest way to ensure that one stays in tune with those whom you purpose to lead. Leadership is (and should be) about service, about ensuring that you understand and reasonably promote the needs and aspirations of those who make the decision (or do not have a choice) but to follow. Being consistent particularly with respect to integrity and ensuring that you practice what you preach enhances success as a leader. In leading adults, respectful communication is also important, and allowing those whom you lead express their opinions safely (without fear of reprimand or humiliation, and without being condescending). It is important to be inclusive when making decisions that will impact the group whilst still ensuring that decisions are in the overall interest of achieving set goals. This will entail being open and transparent and reinforcing expectations and shared objectives. Listening only to opinions or viewpoints that align with yours, and avoiding (or not recognizing, or even misinterpreting) constructive criticism is almost certain to result in failure. A leader must also ensure that he/she is not in competition with those who are being led, as this will limit the perceived usefulness of continuing to follow such a leader.

How do you keep your people open to progress and change?

By staying optimistic, focusing on the 'big picture', and demonstrating through my conduct that it is possible to adapt to challenges, strive to be relevant and make impact despite challenges. I live and practice in an environment that is fraught with numerous persistent challenges that make it difficult to stay focused career-wise. Some of these difficulties sometimes come close to even threatening one's livelihood and career due to sometimes bizarre government policies, and have resulted in a steady out-migration of seemingly scarce qualified neurology (and other specialty) manpower. In-spite of all of these, maintaining an optimistic outlook, but backed by concrete measures to ensuring the continuing professional growth of junior colleagues is crucial. It also requires motivating them and seeking out professional development opportunities for them through one's personal networks.

What were the key characteristics of your best mentor?

My best mentor was consistent and persistent in promoting my career progress, providing inclusive leadership and team work. My progress and success seemed very important to him. Importantly, he did not restrict my desire to explore a sub-specialty area that was different from that in which he was engaged, allowing me to develop my own unique flair. On the contrary, I once had a potential mentor who told me he had *'bigger fish to fry'*. I now realize that although this was in all reality true, it had the potential of scarring a mentee or follower, because it would seem to belittle what, to the person (perceptually) was also important.

Chapter 30
PAL, Pramod K.: Karnataka/India

Bios Dr. Pal is Professor and Head of Neurology at the National Institute of Mental Health and Neurosciences (NIMHANS), Bangalore, India. He studied medicine (MBBS, MD and DM) in India's premier institutions and later specialized in Movement Disorders. He was fortunate to have been mentored by the best in the field—a clinical fellowship in Movement Disorders in University of British Columbia with Dr. Donald B. Calne and a fellowship in Human Motor Physiology and Transcranial Magnetic Stimulation in Toronto with Dr. Robert Chen.

He has been with NIMHANS, an Institute of National Importance for the past 19 years and has helped build a multi-faceted Movement Disorders specialty program which includes a Movement Disorders clinic, Human Motor Physiology laboratory, and a Movement Disorders fellowship program integrated with functional neurosurgery. He mentors students pursuing DM and PhD in Neurology and has more than 225 publications.

He is active across India and Asia Pacific and was, amongst others, Founding Secretary of the Movement Disorders Society of India, Editor-in-Chief of Annals of Movement Disorders. He served on the Education Committees of AOS-MDS and WFN-APRD, and the Editorial Board of the Movement Disorders Journal and PARDS. He is Secretary-Elect of MDS-AOS (2017–2019), Secretary of MDS-AOS (2019–2021) and President-Elect of the Indian Academy of Neurology.

P. K. Pal (✉)
Department of Neurology, National Institute of Mental Health and Neurosciences (NIMHANS), Bangalore, Karnataka, India

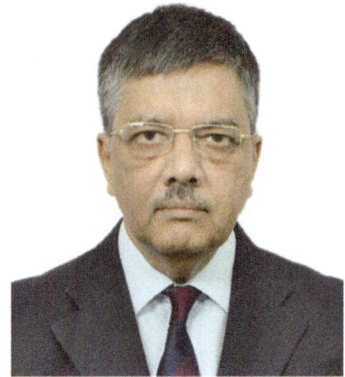

Reprinted with permission from Prof. Pramod Kumar Pal

What motivates you?

I am an optimist and am fortunate to work in my area of interest i.e. Movement Disorders and in an environment that is conducive to pursue a blend of academics, research and patient care. Hope and small successes keep me motivated. The work environment—the team I work with, the facilities available for research and patient care, the projects and the wide range of patients we get to help are definitely key factors. Each time an article from the team gets published or I read about an interesting research and see opportunities to use technology/new methods for investigation, I feel motivated to try harder. I am happy that the zest for learning remains as strong as it was when I started 20 years back.

How do you get others to accept your ideas?

Since I wear many hats, there are numerous occasions where I need to work through to get decisions implemented. I have learnt that early involvement is key to get acceptance. I share ideas early and get inputs so the plans can evolve as we discuss. I ensure that there is a scientific basis to what I suggest and am also practical from an implementation angle. When it involves execution of new ideas, a critical part is to check feasibility and ensure that there are resources/funding/infrastructure and the team is clear with designated roles and responsibilities. At times, if there is no consensus, I try and keep the team together by listening to feedback and ensuring that there are no ad-hoc decisions.

What is the most difficult part of being a leader?

To me, a leader has to keep the team motivated and energized at all times. It is difficult in a set up where the financial rewards are not discretionary based on performance. To overcome this, I use alternatives such as recognizing exceptional work in public meetings, providing opportunities to showcase their work and sharing their achievements in professional social media groups. In large teams, there are very few decisions where there is a complete consensus and this impacts individuals both favorably and adversely. To counter that, I try and balance the work, rewards and opportunities to ensure an equitable and unbiased work environment. This is one of the more difficult issues to address since opportunities are limited.

What advice would you give someone going into a leadership position for the first time?

Leadership is an individual style and you need to find your own. Once you know that, it is important to connect with your team, understand their aspirations and set goals. It is easier to have time bound 30/60/90 day goals that you can set so early milestones are visible. As a first time leader, I would advise you to communicate extensively with your team, peers, and mentors so you are open to feedbacks. Some important points:

1. Give your team the freedom to experiment and grow and celebrate every success.
2. Ensure the work environment is open, fair and rewarding.
3. Stand up for what is right and don't hesitate to be take tough decisions when required.
4. Seek help if required and draw upon seniors and colleagues to get advice.

Chapter 31
POEWE, Werner: Innsbruck/Austria

Bios Professor Werner Poewe is Professor of Neurology and Director of the Department of Neurology at Innsbruck Medical University in Innsbruck, Austria. He held a Residency in Clinical Neurology and Psychiatry at the University of Innsbruck, Austria, from 1977 to 1984. From 1984 to 1985 he teamed up with Gerald Stern and Andrew Lees as a British Council Research Fellow at University College and Middlesex Hospital's Medical School in London to perform clinical studies into levodopa-induced dystonia and pharmacokinetics of levodopa in naïve versus L-Dopa treated Parkinson's disease. Following his return to Austria he held a position as Senior Lecturer in the Department of Neurology at the University of Innsbruck (1986–1989) after which he took over as Professor of Neurology and Acting Director of the Department of Neurology at Virchow Hospital of the Free University of Berlin (1990–1994).

Professor Poewe served as President of the Austrian Society of Neurology from 2002 to 2004 as well as President of the Austrian Parkinson's Disease Society from 1996 to 2009. Professor Poewe served as President of the International Movement Disorder Society from 2000 to 2002, during which period he initiated the creation of important MDS Task Forces related to the critique and development of rating scales and of evidence-based treatment reviews. In his presidency fell the negotiations between the European Section of MDS and the European Federation of Neurological Societies that resulted in formal agreements about joint European congresses. This model served as an important underpinning of the success of the MDS European Section in the past 15 years. Professor Poewe took over as chair of the MDS European Section from 2011 to 2013 and is currently active as member of the Managing Board of the Movement Disorder Scientific Panel of the European Academy of Neurology.

W. Poewe (✉)
Department of Neurology, Medical University Innsbruck, Innsbruck, Austria
e-mail: werner.poewe@i-med.ac.at

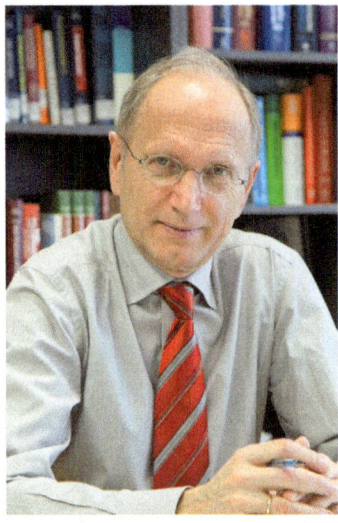

Reprinted with permission from Professor Werner Poewe

What is your greatest strength as a leader?

In trying to answer this sort of question there is always a strong risk of getting it wrong—at least against the gold standard of external judgement by the people you have been working with. Nevertheless, I am happy to confess what I tried to focus on in my leadership roles—regardless how well I did in achieving them. First of all, I have always understood my leadership roles as service to the respective teams which I had to lead. This *primus inter pares* approach to me means creating an environment and atmosphere that will led the individual talents of team members come to their best. To be accepted and successful as a leader, of course, it is essential to have a credible background and uncontested competence in the subject area of an institution (in my case clinical neurology, academic medicine and movement disorders). I am also convinced that one has to set an example in terms of commitment, energy and hard work. Finally, good leaders, I believe, are modest people who know about their limits and who are always ready to listen to the advice of those they are leading.

What do you find, are the most difficult leadership decisions to make?

For me the most difficult decisions to make in leadership is when it comes to bridge a gap between justified but competing interests of individual members or groups within an organization and to then decide on what is best for "the common good" of your organization or team as a whole. These decisions relate to allocation of funds or infrastructure, academic appointments or other types of career moves. It is impossible to please everybody with these decisions, but all the more important to get it right—the latter will not usually be evident until after some time has passed.

A related difficulty is of course always to select between several equally qualified people, when it comes to appointments and also to sometimes having to discontinue or not renew contracts in young people, who have tried their best, but not quite met the expected standards.

What do you like to ask other leaders when you get the chance?

One topic I always like to discuss with other leaders is how they deal with the type of difficult decision points outlined above. I also like to know from others how they find the right balance in allocating time for their leadership duties—most notably those of mentoring young people or the less attractive administrative chores—with their own personal interests in their academic research field. Finally, there are so many common leadership issues in academic institutions and societies across specialties and across the world, that I always try to learn from other leaders how they define their roles in their respective cultural environments and what are the most important priorities to them.

If you could go back and give your 21-year old self a valuable piece of advice, what would that be?

These would be actually three pieces of advice—all of them quite short and simple:

1. Find yourself an academic mentor who you trust and admire.
2. Be sceptical about established "schools of thought" and SOPs.
3. Never strive for applause, and if you get it, ask yourself why.

Chapter 32
POSTUMA, Ron: Montreal/Canada

Bios Dr. Postuma is currently Professor of Neurology at McGill University. A native of Winnipeg, in Canada, he graduated with his Medical Degree from the University of Manitoba. This was followed by a spell as an internal medicine resident, which transitioned to a two-year research fellowship in Alzheimer disease research at the University of Melbourne. During the fellowship, neurology grabbed him, and so he transferred to a Neurology fellowship at McGill University. Wanting to stay in the field of neurodegeneration, but finding Parkinson's disease more satisfying to manage clinically, he chose movement disorders as a subspeciality, and took a fellowship in Movement Disorders at the University of Toronto. He then joined as staff at McGill (getting a Masters in Epidemiology at McGill along the way) and has stayed there since.

His research interests mainly center around non-motor aspects of Parkinson's disease. This includes early detection of PD and other neurodegenerative synucleinopathies, primarily using REM sleep behavior disorder. There is also ongoing work on diagnosis and treatment of sleep disorders in PD, defining subtypes of PD, diagnosis and diagnostic criteria for PD (as part of the Movement Disorders task force on definition of PD), epidemiology of sleep disorders in the general population, and ultimately (hopefully) clinical trials of neuroprotection in the earliest stages of PD. He is also actively involved in teaching, being the previous chair of the Canadian national residents course in movement disorders, and is currently the co-chair of the MDS educational executive committee.

R. Postuma (✉)
Department of Neurology, L7-305 Montreal General Hospital, Montreal, QC, Canada
e-mail: ron.postuma@mcgill.ca

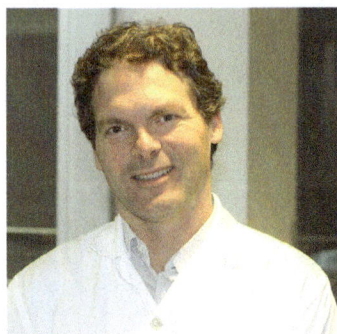

Reprinted with permission from Professor Ron Postuma

How do you build team morale?

People (or at least the kind of people one you want on your team) generally want to be part of something bigger than themselves. Perhaps the best way to build morale is to actively make them part of this bigger thing. Remind everyone of what we are doing and why—show them how their work relates to the broader community and patient care, and keep the big picture and overall goals at the forefront. Also, morale depends upon leading by example. We are social beings; excitement is infectious, as is hard work, as is conscientiousness.

How would you track the performance of your team members and employees? How do you define and measure their success?

My teams are small, so tracking performance is not something formal, but based upon direct contact. Obviously the definition of successful performance depends on the job description. For research students, it's primarily learning and production—how well are they able to complete their projects, how quickly they understand the key concepts, how often I have to explain something, whether they generate next steps on their own, etc. For co-ordinators, it's mostly how smoothly and reliably everything goes—results are gathered accurately and completely, visits don't take too long, minimal patient frustration, etc. For clinical trainees, it's the myriad things that go into being an effective doctor—there are too many of those to list. Overall, the success of one person depends upon many; if the whole team is successful, it is easy to spread the credit.

What motivates you?

Although it's impossible not to be entirely immune to the more prosaic motivational factors (wanting to be recognized for good work, wanting to have an ascending career arc, etc.), I think that there two primary motivators for me. The first is the overall goal of clinical research. Being of a practical mindset, I am less motivated by knowledge for knowledge's sake than by the desire to feel my work will change something concrete. I eventually want to be part of a major advance in clinical care; not necessarily the one who did it all, but at least a useful cog in the machine. The second thing that motivates me is the fun of the research process itself; planning the studies, thinking of all the angles and possible outcomes, getting everything operationalized, and then (best of all) seeing the results for the first time. Having a spreadsheet in front of me containing a blizzard of study results, with my job now is to make sense of it all—that is work-heaven for me.

Who inspires/d you and why?

For me, it's not just one person. I've had terrific mentors (e.g. training with Tony Lang was wonderful), and many people over the years have steered me in the right direction. Mostly, I find that I take a little from everyone; there's the supervisor from residency who provided to a patient an explanation of neurodegeneration which has now became my standard explanation of Parkinson's disease, the patient who said something that stuck with me forever, the idea I got from a random lecturer on a seemingly-unrelated topic, the colleagues who keep my standards up, and my family who keeps me happy and grounded.

Chapter 33
SINGLETON, Andrew: Maryland/USA

Bios Andrew Singleton received his B.Sc. from the University of Sunderland, UK and his Ph.D. from the University of Newcastle upon Tyne, UK. His postdoctoral studies were spent at the Mayo Clinic in Jacksonville Florida. He then moved to the National Institute on Aging at NIH Bethesda, MD. In 2008 he became the Chief of the Laboratory of Neurogenetics, and in 2016 he was named an NIH Distinguished Investigator. He has published more than 550 articles on a wide variety of topics. His laboratory comprises ~60 staff, including six principal investigators and three group leaders, working on the genetic basis of neurological disorders including Parkinson's disease, Alzheimer's disease, dystonia, ataxia, dementia with Lewy bodies, and amyotrophic lateral sclerosis.

He currently serves on the scientific advisory board of the Lewy Body Dementia Association. Andrew has won numerous prestigious awards including the Boehringer Mannheim Research Award, the NIH Director's Award twice, the Annemarie Opprecht Award for Parkinson's disease research, the Jay van Andel Award for Outstanding Achievement in Parkinson's Disease Research, and the American Academy of Neurology Movement Disorders Award. Andrew was recently a proud recipient of an honorary doctorate from his alma mater, the University of Sunderland.

A. Singleton (✉)
Laboratory of Neurogenetics, NIA IRP NIH, Bethesda, MD, USA
e-mail: singleta@mail.nih.gov

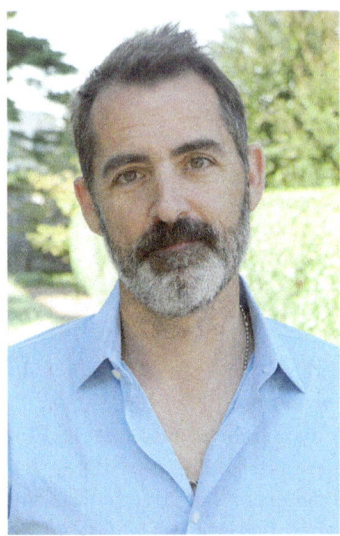

Reprinted with permission from Dr. Andrew Singleton

How did you become a leader in your field?

Whatever I am I didn't get there by myself. My mentors were a huge help, first Chris Morris while I was in Newcastle upon Tyne, then John Hardy while I was at the Mayo Clinic and my early years here at NIH. They gave me the room to try things, gave me more opportunity than I probably deserved, and also made it their job to promote me to the outside world. Being in genetics in the late 90's through to 2010 also proved to be wonderful timing—the huge wins that could be made in that era could still be accomplished by single labs, or small groups. The same is not true anymore.

Who inspires/d you and why?

To the truest meaning of the word inspiration—I would say patients. I don't meet patients as regularly as I would like, however, there are a few that have really touched me, particularly those from families that have been devastated by disease. When someone is looking to you to help provide an answer for their family it's pretty strong stuff. These experiences have made me both want to do more and regret any wasted time or effort. If I were to change the wording of this question from 'inspire' to 'drive'—I would say a driver for me is not knowing something. I hate not knowing something, so I am driven to try to understand.

How would you deliver bad news to your team?

Quickly and with transparency. I think you have to be direct and clear while at the same time having compassion. Then you have to give folks time to process, the ability to ask questions, and sometimes (and after a long enough time) a nudge to move forward. As trite as it might sound my default is always to see if there is a way to find a positive in the situation, or at least solutions to moving forward and dealing with the problem.

When do you consider partnering with others, what factors are deal-breakers for you? How do you balance partnership and competition in science?

This is hugely important in the work I do. My main rule is "don't work with assholes" and this seems to be pretty effective. Working with good people, such as those in IPDGC, makes collaborating a joy. Balancing partnership and competition is extremely difficult. Large consortia can lead to a monopoly that doesn't necessarily have the urgency it should. In this regard you just need leaders within that group that keep pushing for the next step forward, and giving the up and coming folks the space to take responsibility for leading things.

How do you lead through change?

The first thing to recognize is that whatever the change, even apparently positive, it always evokes a certain amount of worry. In some ways dealing with change is the same as dealing with bad news, I believe you have to present the facts, allow people to question (which, frankly often raises interesting ideas and questions I hadn't considered), and then chart a path forward. I think it's also important, if you have to change in some way that is not necessarily your choice, not to undermine the change, it just ultimately leads to discontent.

How do you get others to accept your ideas?

By explaining the reasoning behind the idea. It's important to realize that the underlying reasons for a decision or an idea are often quite complex, involving a longer term vision, or a series of experiences. I think by explaining that reasoning you achieve a few things, most notably you get buy in, but perhaps more importantly it is a teaching moment where you get to present the big picture, the non-obvious (sometimes political) influencers, and any long term vision you may have. This gives power to those working with you, and the potential to contribute beyond their initial task.

Chapter 34
STANDAERT, David G.: Alabama/USA

Bios Dr. Standaert came to the field of movement disorders in a deliberate way, but it has grown in to a passion. He was interested in science early; inspired by his father, a pharmacologist, he started working in research labs when he was about 14 years old. At Harvard College, he studied biochemistry and worked on projects related to motor control, studying *Homerus americanus* (the American lobster) with Ed Kravitz. He went to Washington University in St. Louis in 1982 to pursue a combined MD/PhD degree. His thesis mentors were Clifford Saper, then a new assistant professor of Neurology, and Philip Needleman, Chair of the Department of Pharmacology. Dr. Standaert launched his PhD work just as Phil was discovering the atrial natriuretic peptide (ANP) in the heart (he preferred to call it "atriopeptin," but that name never caught on). Clif and he looked for it in the brain, and they were amazed to find that this hormone from the heart was also in brain neurons involved in cardiovascular regulation. This was a very hot topic of the time, and led to a wild scientific ride.

Dr. Standaert's clinical neurology training started at the University of Pennsylvania. Towards the end of residency, he was actively searching for a path forward that would let him combine his interests in brain structure and chemistry with hands-on clinical skills. Inspired largely by Howard Hurtig and Matt Stern, the leaders of the movement disorders group at Penn, he applied for a fellowship with Anne Young and Jack Penney who were then at the University of Michigan and well known for their work on basal ganglia pathways. Before he could join the lab, Anne was appointed Chief of Neurology at the Massachusetts General Hospital (MGH). Dr. Standaert started his fellowship at MGH in 1992. Over the next 14 years, he built both his clinic and research careers at MGH, seeing patients in the outpatient clinic and developing a bench laboratory research program.

In 2006, he was recruited to the University of Alabama at Birmingham (UAB) by Ray Watts, then Chair of the Department of Neurology. The idea was simple but inspiring: UAB wanted to build a new translational research group in neurodegenerative disease, and was looking for a leader. His family and he made a leap of faith,

---

D. G. Standaert (✉)
Department of Neurology, University of Alabama at Birmingham, Birmingham, AL, USA
e-mail: dstandaert@uabmc.edu

moving from Boston to Birmingham, Alabama to build this program. Over the first 5 years, he recruited the faculty for what became the Center for Neurodegeneration and Experimental Therapeutics (CNET), now a very successful group of 11 laboratories with more than 80 faculty, students and staff. In 2010, Dr. Watts became the Dean at UAB (and later the President of UAB). Dr. Standaert was appointed Chair of the Department of Neurology in 2011, and now leads a group of about 80 faculty and more than 300 residents, students, and staff. He also has a number of other leadership roles, serving on hospital boards, as a member of the National Institute of Neurological Disorders and Stroke (NINDS) Board of Scientific Counselors, and as Associate Editor for *Movement Disorders*.

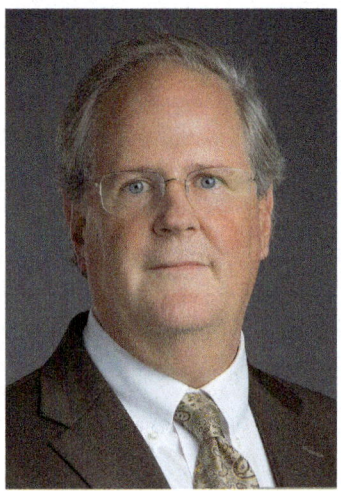

Reprinted with permission from Dr. David G. Standaert

Are leaders born or made?

A tough question, and as a scientist I would first acknowledge that all I have is opinion, as there are no adequately controlled experiments addressing the question. My belief is that they are largely "made," but the process starts very early. I think the most crucial element is mentorship. In my case, I grew up in a household where my father was Chair of a department of pharmacology (at Georgetown), and my early memories are of his efforts to build the program, recruiting faculty (many of whom became life-long friends of the family) and renovating space (one consequence of this was that my childhood bedroom was furnished in cast-off laboratory benches and cabinets). Later, I worked with Clif Saper, who for the last 27 years has been Chair of Neurology at Beth Israel in Boston, and Anne Young, the first woman to serve as a Chief of Service in the history of MGH. Given these origins, it seems no accident that I have also ended up as a department chair.

My more recent experiences, however, have made me aware that history and experiences alone are not enough. Effective leadership takes more conscious effort than I anticipated. I have found a need to be deliberate and thoughtful about in deciding which issues I should engage on, and which are best left undecided for the present or delegated to others. I have also learned how critical it is to assemble an effective support team. In retrospect, I can see that my mentors did this as well, but at the time it happened so seamlessly that I did not appreciate how difficult this can be.

How can a leader fail?

I think leaders fail when they don't recognize that you can't lead anything alone. To be a leader, you must have followers. I have found it useful to think about why people might follow my lead. Sometimes, they may follow because it is simply a rule of some kind (follow or you will be fired!). In my experience, this works at best only transiently. There may be occasional situations where this is the right approach with a specific person and situation, but over the long term is usually not successful. A much better situation is when you can convince others to follow because you explain to them that you are leading them to a better place or outcome. Perhaps you are reorganizing work assignments for a large group of people; the change may be disruptive, but if you can explain how the outcome will be better for all there is a good chance that they will let you lead them to this new situation. The most powerful form of leadership, however, is when you can convince people to follow you even though the outcome is uncertain. This involves building faith: when your followers trust you sufficiently, they will let you lead (at least for a while) even without understanding exactly where they are going.

How do you lead through change?

In healthcare, we are constantly in a state of change. This is driven in part by the politics and economics of how we provide care, but also by discovery which is constantly changing our understanding of disease and the methods we have to care for people. There is also the human element of change in an academic environment, with constant turnover of students and residents and the natural progression of faculty through the academic ranks.

I have had the most success with change when there is an opportunity to build consensus around the issue. When there are important changes anticipated, bringing together a representative group to discuss the issue and solutions can be powerful. Even if the change is externally imposed and the alternatives are few, having the opportunity to consider the effects as a group can accelerate acceptance.

The opposite is also true, that without consensus change can be hard. I often find that people are putting up with problems that should not be allowed to continue, simply because they feel that change is not possible. It may be difficult to change a complex system because of one voice of complaint—but if we can come together around a common solution, then that can be a powerful force for change.

While I emphasize the value of consensus, this does not mean that I favor a democratic approach. Indeed, while I try to gather viewpoints from many and I hope to lead everyone to a shared vision, I would almost never subject an important decision to a vote of any kind. At least in my current roles, I think as leader I am charged with owning the final decision and that vote counting would in most cases be more of an obstacle to change than a help.

If you could go back and give your 21-year old self a valuable piece of advice, what would you say?

When I was 21, I was still in college and had the idea that I wanted to pursue science and do something important. Looking back, I still admire the goal but I think that the means of accomplishing it are different than I imagined. I think that in the intervening 37 years, I have done two things that turned out to be really valuable. One is that I made a commitment to caring for and working with patients with movement disorders. Over the years, I have seen many thousands of patients with Parkinson disease and other conditions. I feel I have helped many individually, and the projects I have been engaged in have helped many more on a systematic level. Many of these patients have become friends and partners over the years. The other important thing that I have done is to engage in training and mentorship of students, residents and fellows. There have been a lot—I have trained more than 25 movement disorders fellows, a similar number of postdocs, about a dozen graduate students, and many more medical students, residents, and others. I have learned that this is an exponential process, as each of these individuals gives rise to their own intellectual descendants. Both of these goals have developed over time, but I think if I had understood how important they would become, I might have moved more deliberately towards engagement with patients and trainees earlier in my career.

Chapter 35
STERN, Matthew B.: Pennsylvania/USA

Bios Matthew B. Stern, MD, is the Parker Family Professor Emeritus of Neurology at the Perelman School of Medicine at the University of Pennsylvania and Director Emeritus of the Parkinson's Disease and Movement Disorders Center.

Dr. Stern received his B.A. from Harvard University and medical degree from Duke University in Durham, North Carolina. He completed his training in neurology at the University of Pennsylvania.

Dr. Stern cofounded Penn's Parkinson's Disease and Movement Disorders Center, which he helped build into one of the premier centers of its kind in the world. Dr. Stern has authored or co-authored numerous papers on Parkinson's disease (PD) and related disorders and edited and/or co-edited 8 books. Dr. Stern has been principal investigator or co-principal investigator of many studies related to PD and movement disorders. He was also co-chair of VA Cooperative Study 468 investigating Deep Brain Stimulation in Parkinson's disease and founding director of the Philadelphia VA Parkinson's Disease Research, Education and Clinical Center. He serves on numerous consulting boards and has lectured throughout the world. He is an inaugural member of Penn's Academy of Master Clinicians and is a Past President of the International Parkinson and Movement Disorder Society which has awarded him its President's Distinguished Service Award and Honorary Membership. The University of Pennsylvania recently established the Howard Hurtig-Matthew Stern Professorship in Neurology to commemorate his contributions to Penn Medicine.

M. B. Stern (✉)
Perelman School of Medicine, University of Pennsylvania, Philadelphia, PA, USA
e-mail: mbstern@pennmedicine.upenn.edu

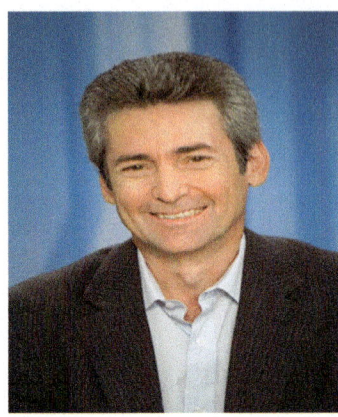

Reprinted with permission from Professor Matthew B. Stern

What steps do you take to resolve complicated leadership problems?

As in any negotiation, resolving problems as a leader depends upon understanding the give and take involved in any successful arbitration. Complicated leadership issues often involve conflict resolution. The parties involved in any conflict need to feel heard so listening is a key quality of any successful leader. Regardless of an immediate sense of resolution, a leader should take a day or two to consider options and present a resolution that reflects careful thought and compromise. Above all, successful leaders must separate their own career objectives and egos from their charges. They must judge their own success through the accomplishments of their faculty and staff. That attitude alone will ease the burden of complicated issues that always involve interpersonal challenges. Knowing that a leader is genuinely interested in the success and comfort of their faculty and staff engenders the trust and respect necessary to be an effective leader.

What is one mistake you witness leaders making more frequently than others?

The one mistake that seems to recur among academic and clinical leaders is self-interest. When leaders elevate their own agendas and their own career advancement above those of their staff, they will inevitably exacerbate conflict and lose respect. Even the most senior leaders often have difficulty sacrificing a speaking or publishing opportunity rather than recommending that they be replaced as speaker or first author by a younger colleague. Academic advancement within one's institution is often at odds with effective leadership qualities, especially when even the most senior members of a faculty are judged by their academic productivity. However, the responsibility of effective leadership is first and foremost to be a trusted mentor. The most effective leaders produce successful clinical and academic "offspring". These individuals are a reflection of the leader and mentor who guided them and should be the major criteria by which leaders judge themselves.

What are the challenges for a young scientist/academic/ clinician today compared to the past and how to tackle them?

The challenges inherent in an academic and/or clinical career today are an accentuation of issues we all faced along the way. Funding is tighter, the clinical environment more regimented and competition for advancement more intense. Where my career goal was to be a clinician, educator and investigator, today's young neurologists are often faced with deciding which path to pursue in order to succeed. As a mentor, a leader is often in the delicate role of steering a young career and guiding a young person to ensure success. It is critical for leaders to reassure their younger staff and faculty that success is measured in many ways so a failure to succeed at raising research funds does not lessen one's potential as an outstanding clinician and educator. Part of a leader's responsibility is to recognize the strengths and weaknesses in young academicians and clinicians and value the heterogeneity of talent. Finally, young academicians and clinicians should identify role models and mentors who will help them adapt to the changing landscape of clinical and academic medicine. A good mentor often makes the difference between a stalled career and a satisfying and rewarding path to success.

What do you like to ask other leaders when you get the chance?

One of the real pleasures of a career with colleagues around the globe is the chance to convene, socialize and share insights into today's leadership challenges. While every leader has a different leadership "style", most are dealing with similar leadership and administrative issues. I have found it helpful to ask colleagues how they balance their roles as clinician, mentor, scientist and administrator. I am particularly interested in how leaders delegate responsibilities to allow them adequate time to mentor and "lead". What kind of administrative staff have they found most effective in dealing with institutional oversight so that communication is effective, work flow is efficient and time spent in less impactful and meaningful pursuits is minimized? Being open to change is one of the most desirable attributes a leader can possess and learning from colleagues is often the spark that fuels innovation and novel initiatives.

Chapter 36
SUE, Carolyn: Sydney/Australia

Bios Carolyn Sue is currently appointed as Head of the Department of Neurogenetics and the Executive Director of the Kolling Institute at Royal North Shore Hospital, University of Sydney. She was the first female adult neurologist to be promoted to Professor in Australia and is the inaugural Professor in Neurology at Royal North Shore Hospital. Professor Sue trained in the field of movement disorders with Professor John Morris and continued her post-doctoral studies at Columbia University, New York, USA. Dr. Sue's research interests are focused on two main areas: the role of mitochondrial function in neurodegenerative disease and the genetics of movement disorders. Dr. Sue founded the Familial Parkinson's Disease Research Clinic at Royal North Shore Hospital, and has spear-headed national collaborative genetic studies in Parkinson's disease. Her research group has established the use of patient derived stem cell models to investigate the pathophysiology underlying neurological disease and has identified new therapeutic approaches to prevent the neurodegenerative process in Parkinson's disease.

Dr. Sue is a Founding Director of the Australian Mitochondrial Disease Foundation and is currently appointed to the International Parkinson and Movement Disorder Society's Task Force on Genetic Nomenclature in Movement Disorders and the Faculty of the LEAP program. She is also Chair of the Clinical Trials Network for the Movement Disorder Society of Australia and New Zealand and appointed to the Scientific Advisory Committee of Parkinson's NSW. She has previously been appointed to the Scientific Issues committee and as Treasurer (Asian Oceanic Section), of the International Parkinson and Movement Disorder Society.

C. M. Sue (✉)
Executive Director, Kolling Institute, University of Sydney and Royal North Shore Hospital, Northern Sydney Local Health District, Sydney, NSW, Australia
e-mail: carolyn.sue@sydney.edu.au

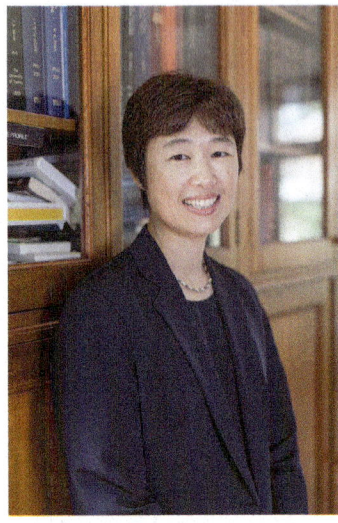

Reprinted with permission from Dr. Carolyn Sue

As an organization gets larger there can be a tendency for the "institution" to dampen the "inspiration". How do you keep this from happening?

I look to my patients for my inspiration; it is for them that I strive for excellence in my clinical and academic pursuits. I consider it a privilege to be involved in their care and to have the opportunity to help improve their lives. Patients always know what medical problems need to be solved- we just have to listen and interpret what they say. If enthusiasm is dampened by the growth of an organization, I think about what is in the best interest of the patient, and this keeps my focus on what is most important. This attitude is characteristic of my whole team and we help each other to keep this goal foremost in our minds.

What are a few resources you would recommend to someone looking to gain insight into becoming a better leader?

I mainly draw on the experience and advice of those I respect and admire. Having multiple mentors who are happy to give constructive advice is important to me. I like to learn as much as I can from as many people as I can. Having wise senior advisors is crucial, and in addition to this, I have found that seeking input from those who follow you as a leader is also vital to becoming a better leader. Being involved in our Movement Disorders Society's LEAP program has definitely provided a formal structure to how I think about leadership and I would highly recommend this program as a resource for those who would like to become better leaders. I would definitely recommend interactions with the LEAP Faculty as well as the LEAPers from each course to gain insights into better leadership principles.

How do you deal with disagreement within your team?

Disagreement is best dealt with quickly and as constructively as possible. Having clarity about what we are trying to do and reflecting on why we are trying to achieve it helps to keep my team unified and centered on our shared vision and common goals. We try to keep the lines of communication open within the whole team. If there is disagreement along the way, this is usually due to varying perspectives, a misunderstanding or a miscommunication. If this situation arises, I think it best that we try to address it early and transparently, so that we can seek resolution as early as possible.

Do you have advice addressed to young females in their early career?

I would encourage young females who are early in their career to enjoy and embrace both the professional and personal aspects of their life. Work-life balance is difficult for many and most of us struggle to achieve a good balance, regardless of the stage of our career or gender. I would advise young females who are early in their careers to pursue excellence at all times, have the confidence to back themselves and stand up for what they know is equal and right. Building a support network of like-minded people around you is helpful as is staying focused on what you would like to achieve.

Chapter 37
TABRIZI, Sarah J.: London/UK

Bios Sarah Tabrizi graduated in biochemistry then medicine from the University of Edinburgh in 1992. She's worked on research into neurodegenerative diseases since her PhD at UCL 1996–1999. After her clinical training, she obtained a DH National Clinician Scientist Fellowship in 2002 to work on protein misfolding at UCL. She was promoted to Senior Lecturer and Honorary Consultant Neurologist in 2003, and to Full Professor in 2009. In 2016, she founded the UCL Huntington's Disease Centre where she is currently the Director and was appointed joint Head of the UCL Department of Neurodegenerative Disease in 2017. Sarah's research focuses on understanding the basic cellular mechanisms of neurodegeneration, in particular Huntington's disease and finding effective disease-modifying treatments for this disorder. Sarah was global clinical PI on the world's first gene-silencing study of Huntington's disease using anti-sense oligonucleotide therapy, sponsored by Ionis pharmaceuticals, the safety study for which successfully completed in December 2017. Sarah co-founded the UK All Party Parliamentary Group for HD in 2010, was elected a Fellow of the UK Academy of Medical Sciences in 2014 and in 2017, she received the seventh Leslie Gehry Brenner Prize for Innovation in Science awarded by the Hereditary Disease Foundation.

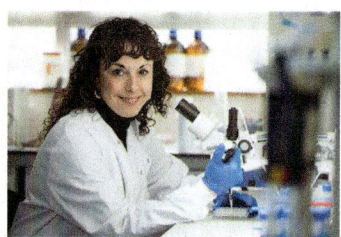

Reprinted with permission from Prof. Sarah Tabrizi

S. Tabrizi (✉)
Department of Neurodegenerative Disease, Huntington's Disease Centre, UCL Institute of Neurology, National Hospital for Neurology and Neurosurgery, London, UK
e-mail: s.tabrizi@ucl.ac.uk

What was the best advice you ever received in your early/late career?

The best advice I received in my early career was to do a medical degree after my science degree in biochemistry that allowed me to combine basic science with clinical research. The best advice I got in my later career was to make sure that I focused and that if I really wanted to find an effective treatment for Huntington's disease that I was best to just focus on Huntington's disease and nothing else.

Did you ever consider leaving the career path you were on in order to doing something different (completely else or somewhat related)?

No, never. I am very focused!

What influenced you to stay and keep going?

I am passionate about finding a treatment for Huntington's disease. I have been seeing patients for twenty-two years doing regular Huntington's disease clinics and being close to such a devastating disease and the patients and families means that you are completely dedicated to finding an effective treatment for this terrible disease.

What does Neurology mean to you? (i.e., job/hobby/inner calling/passion/destiny)?

Well I am passionate about my research and also my work on trying to find treatments for Huntington's disease. When I give advice to my mentees or to future students, I always say that I think it's important to be passionate about what you do at work as it takes up so much of your life. I also think that it's important to try and have fun at the same time and to train the next generation of future leaders.

What advice would you give a young talented neurologist/movement disorder expert?

Learn coping strategies to become resilient because it's important for survival to cope with paper and grant rejections. Focus and tenacity—never give up, believe in what you are doing and develop a passion and try and be as nice as you can be. It does help, but don't let yourself be kicked around! Try and make your work as much fun as possible because you need to enjoy it. Important to always keep seeing patients as they keep you grounded and they're motivating. Always ask for advice and mentoring as you need it and try and inspire and mentor the next generation and finally, never forget your loved ones—they really are the most important people in your life!

How did you become a leader in your field?

I suppose a combination of hard work and being passionate about what I do.

Chapter 38
TAKAHASHI, Ryosuke: Kyoto/Japan

My Advice to Young Colleagues

Bios Ryosuke Takahashi, MD, PhD graduated from Kyoto University, Japan in 1983. He completed his neurology residency in Kyoto University Hospital and its affiliated hospitals and worked as a staff neurologist at Tokyo Metropolitan Neurological Hospital. In 1989, he started basic researches on neurodegenerative disorders and neuronal apoptosis as a staff scientist at Tokyo Metropolitan Institute for Neurosciences, then he worked as a postdoctoral fellow with Prof. John C. Reed at the Burnham Institute, California, USA. He became Laboratory Head at RIKEN Brain Science Institute, Japan, in 1999. In 2005, he was appointed Professor and Chair of Neurology at Kyoto University Hospital and Kyoto University Graduate School of Medicine. He served as the chair of the task force for 2011 version of the treatment guidelines for Parkinson' s disease in Japan. From 2014 to 2018, he served as the President of Japanese Society of Neurology. He also serves as the Vice President of Japanese Society for Neuroscience. He is on the editorial board of *Movement Disorders*, *Journal of Neural Transmission, and Molecular Brain*. He has published more than 300 original and review articles in peer-reviewed international journals including *Nature*, *Cell*, *Neuron*, *Nature Genetics*, *Nature Neuroscience* and *Annals of Neurology*.

His major research interests are the molecular pathogenetic mechanisms underlying Parkinson's disease and related disorders and development of disease-modifying therapies against neurodegenerative disorders.

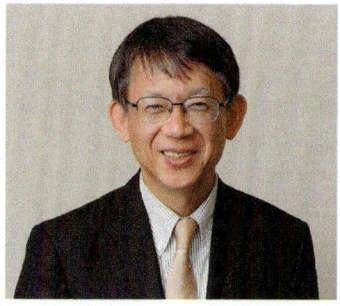

R. Takahashi (✉)
Department of Neurology, Kyoto University Graduate School of Medicine, Kyoto, Japan
e-mail: ryosuket@kuhp.kyoto-u.ac.jp

What advice would you give a young talented neurologist/movement disorder expert?

If you have a big dream, the goal is distant and it is hard to keep motivation. You may be depressed when the goal looks too far away. Enjoy small successes in your daily life.

Believe that a big success is obtained based on accumulation of small successes of everyday life.

What is your greatest strength as a leader?

A leader should have a high ability to share her/his dreams with the members of her/his group. I am good at convincing my colleagues how important it is to reach the goal and encouraging them to strive hard for it.

How can a leader fail?

A leader should have a clear vision about the future of the society and a strong determination to realize it. But a clear vision is not enough. If she/he does not listen to the opinions of other people who has a different thought from her/him, she/he may lose balanced view on complicated issues. Before making a difficult decision, the leader should be very open-minded.

Would you do differently if you could start over?

When I was a high school student, I like to read novels. My bookshelf was full of books of Japanese novels and essays. I once dreamed of being a literary critic instead of a medical doctor. However, I am an extremely slow writer. If I become a critic, I should have always suffered from keeping the deadline. So I am happy with my real life, although I often worry about the deadline for manuscripts.

Chapter 39
TANNER, Caroline: California/USA

Bios Caroline M. Tanner, MD, PhD, FAAN, is the Director of the Parkinson's Disease Research, Education and Clinical Center at the San Francisco Veterans Affairs Health Care System and Professor in the Department of Neurology, University of California, San Francisco. Her clinical practice specializes in movement disorders. Her research interests include investigations of the descriptive epidemiology, environmental and genetic determinants, biomarkers and early detection of movement disorders and neurodegenerative diseases. Dr. Tanner and her colleagues have identified associations between exposures including certain pesticides, solvents and persistent environmental pollutants and increased risk of Parkinson's disease, and a greater risk in individuals with certain genetic variants (gene-environment interaction). She is the principal investigator of the online Fox Insight study, and co-principal investigator of a large interventional study using telemedicine. Dr. Tanner is past co-chair of the Parkinson Study Group (PSG); she serves on the Scientific Advisory Boards of the Michael J. Fox Foundation and the National Spasmodic Dysphonia Association, on the Linked Clinical Trials Committee of the Cure Parkinson's Trust, and on committees for NIH and the American Academy of Neurology (AAN). Her honors include the AAN Movement Disorders Research Award in 2012 and the White House Champions of Change for Parkinson's in 2015.

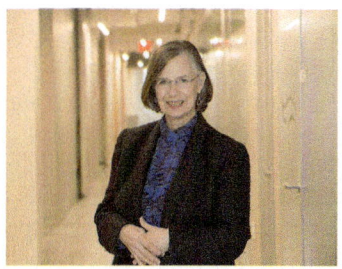

C. M. Tanner (✉)
Movement Disorders and Neuromodulation Center, Department of Neurology, Weill Institute for Neurosciences, University of California - San Francisco, San Francisco, CA, USA

Parkinson's Disease Research Education and Clinical Center, San Francisco Veteran's Affairs Health Care System, San Francisco, CA, USA
e-mail: CAROLINE.TANNER@UCSF.EDU

© Springer Nature Switzerland AG 2019
S. A. Schneider, C. Comella (eds.), *Leadership in Movement Disorders*,
https://doi.org/10.1007/978-3-030-12967-5_39

What do you like about managing and leading people?

I love learning about the many wonderful characteristics in each team member, and creatively using those to develop the strongest possible team. Each person brings a fascinating array of strengths and weaknesses. The trick is to enhance the strengths and minimize the weaknesses. Assembling the right combination of team members can be magical. Assigning tasks to take advantage of individual talents, giving constructive direction and rewarding success all contribute to a positive team dynamic. Respect and appreciation of each team member is foundational. When the chemistry is right, everyone is a leader. We all learn from one another. Each team member's creativity is maximized, and our work is much stronger.

Where do the great ideas come from in your organization?

The best ideas are attuned to our core values. They come from the heart, as well as the mind. All of the best ideas are a team product. An idea sparks in one team member, and that begets another spark in a second team member, and so on, until ultimately we are shining a light into a former area of darkness. Our patients are the best source of inspiration.

How do you communicate the "core values" to your team? How do you ensure your team and its activities are aligned with your "core values"?

Our core values are best communicated by example. By acting in accordance with these values, our work environment embodies them.
How do you deal with disagreement within your team?
When there is a significant disagreement, it is best to understand clearly each person's point of view. Often, this requires meeting individually with each person, and listening deeply. Much of the time, both individuals have a valid point, and the task is to understand the best way to take the good aspects from each. In the best circumstances, the two team members who disagree will work together to resolve the conflict. Usually this resolution is a better solution.

How would you deliver bad news to your team? How did you a handle a time when you had to make an unpopular decision?

Honest, respectful communication of bad news is key. Truthfully letting people know what is happening can reduce fear and anxiety, even when the news is bad. Gossip and speculation can magnify the bad news and cause a lot of unnecessary sorrow. It is useful to have a team meeting, so that everyone hears the same information, can ask questions and hear answers. It is important to be available to people, to listen to people and to understand their concerns. When it is possible to respond positively to even a few concerns, doing so is very helpful. If it is possible to ask people for advice or assistance in addressing the reasons for the bad news, or to allow them some aspects of choice or autonomy, damage can be minimized.

What were the key characteristics of your best mentor?

My mentor recognized potential in me, and, quite amazingly, simply believed that I would succeed. My mentor treated me as an intellectual peer, albeit one with much less experience. My mentor provided opportunities, and then stepped back and allowed me to take responsibility. My mentor was available when I needed help. My mentor delighted in my success.

Chapter 40
TRENKWALDER, Claudia: Kassel/Germany

Bios Claudia Trenkwalder, MD, started her clinical education in neurology and movement disorders at the Dept. Neurology of the University Hospital in Munich in 1988, was head of the "Movement Disorders and Sleep" research group at the Max-Planck Institute of Psychiatry in Munich from 1993 to 2000, before moving to the University Medical Center of Goettingen. Since 2003 she is Medical Director of the Paracelsus-Elena Klinik, in Kassel, and since 2012, she is Full Professor of Neurology as a Foundation Chair at Dept. of Neurosurgery, University Medical Center Goettingen, Germany.

She has published more than 380 peer reviewed papers and is currently President-Elect of International Parkinson Disease and Movement Disorder Society, and was President of the World Association of Sleep Medicine (WASM) from 2011 to 2013 and active member of many national and international scientific societies.

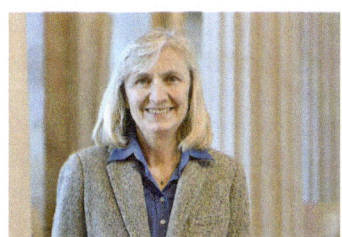

Reprinted with permission from Prof. Claudia Trenkwalder

C. Trenkwalder (✉)
Paracelsus-Elena Hospital, Kassel, Germany

Department of Neurosurgery, University Medical Center Goettingen, Kassel, Germany

Do you have advice for young women in the early stages of their career?

Young women should not be hindered by thoughts related to being a woman, instead they should start their career by simply pursuing the work they like doing. If they are interested in clinical work, organizing patient care or hospitals, that's fine—do it! Success can be achieved in many ways and in many areas. Whatever area you are in, however, it needs a lot of work, more than the usual 8 h at the beginning, and that applies to both men and women! Most importantly, however, is the question about family: do not choose your area of expertise, your clinical or research career in anticipation of your future roles as a wife, mother and center of a family. You never know what will happen… maybe the ideal partner and future co-parent is not around, or you become pregnant at the "wrong" moment! My advice is that all kinds of work are compatible with having a family—you will make the right decisions when the time comes. While it is true that there are better or worse solutions in combining a career and kids, you really have to like what you do, otherwise it will never work and you will be unfulfilled and resentful: if you want to be a neurosurgeon and enjoy it, then you will find a solution otherwise you will be bored senseless if you instead choose to work in a lab from 8–5 in order to accommodate a future hypothetical family.

What advice would you give someone going into a leadership position for the first time?

If someone starts to chair a research group, for example, it is very important to become really knowledgeable about the topic, the content, the literature, the possible projects, anything, that relates to the position. To be knowledgeable gives you self-confidence and strengthens your position without forcing it. Your colleagues will automatically perceive this, and you can let them have discussions—but be one step ahead, read the most recent literature thoroughly, think about a new project and get advice from different areas such as statistics, ethics, and basic science etc. Tell your colleagues frankly, but respectfully, what you want to achieve and make your leadership role clear. Try to assign people to tasks they can really accomplish, avoid defining visions and goals that are unlikely to be fulfilled. Be realistic—and leave some topics for discussion, let your colleagues come up with their ideas. Don't be shy—now, you are on your way to being a leader, you need to behave like one—and you won't believe it, but you also have to dress like one!

What is your greatest strength as a leader?

My greatest strength—in my view—is, that I am really interested in people: in the big and wonderful diversity of humans, of their different cultures, talents and ways of working. I like to listen to people, to observe them—I am not primarily a talker.

Therefore, I am able to better find out what peoples' talents and strengths are. I am quite flexible in building groups and assigning tasks to colleagues. It is great fun to see how someone suddenly becomes very successful, if you assign him or her to a very different task. For example, I assigned one of our doctors, who came from Russia, to control encoding diagnoses and therefore taking responsibility of our hospital's economy. He increased our revenue substantially when combining his medical knowledge with this economical talent. You can find such opportunities all over, you only have to look for them and use them. I do not look for conflicts, I prefer communicating in a nice way, which encourages young people to go their individual way and find success!

What was the best advice you ever received in your early/late career?

The best advice was: Don't think about leadership, just work continuously the best you can, and you will get there! This may not be true in all areas, but it applies a lot in research and clinics. Today, you have to know the inside of your chosen career path in order to obtain grants, to find mentors and opportunities, and to join societies. Another piece of good advice was: Better to sit next to a VIP for one evening at dinner as opposed to writing emails and making phone calls to reach out to them. Many of my career steps were built by just talking to people personally about my research or work—these are the bonds that help most and last the longest. At the very first MDS Congress, back in 1990, my mentor bought me a dinner ticket and told me to sit next to the most important man, and talk to him! It worked!

Chapter 41
TRUONG, Daniel: California/USA

Bios Dr. Daniel Truong graduated from the medical school at Ludwig Albert University in Freiburg, Germany, followed by fellowships in Movement Disorders at Columbia University in New York and the prestigious National Hospital for Nervous Disease at Queen Square, London, UK, studying under two of the founders of the field, Professor Stanley Fahn and the late Prof. David Marsdens. He was the first neurologist to arrive in Southern California with formal fellowship training in Parkinson's disease and Movement Disorders. He was previously the medical director of the American Parkinson Disease Association Information and Referral Center in Orange County and Long Beach.

Dr. Truong was the founder of the Parkinson's and Movement Disorders program at the University of California, Irvine and left in 1997 to form the Parkinson and Movement Disorder Institute. He is also founder of the National Spasmodic Dysphonia Association, for which he served as chairman of the medical advisory board from 1990 to 1997. He is the current President of the International Association for Parkinsonism and Related Disorders and Editor of the new journal, *Clinical Parkinsonism Related Disorders*.

President, International Association of Parkinsonism and Related Disorders www.iaprd.org.

Editor in Chief: Clinical Parkinsonism and Related Disorders.

Associate Editor: Journal of Neurological Sciences; Consulting Editor: eNS.

Editorial Board: Parkinsonism Related Disorders; Journal of Neural Transmission.

D. Truong (✉)
Department of Neurosciences, UC Riverside, Riverside, CA, USA

The Parkinson and Movement Disorder Institute, Fountain Valley, CA, USA
http://www.pmdi.org/dr-daniel-truong.html

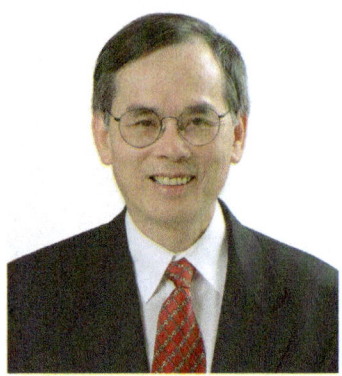

What are you most proud of with regards to your career achievements and development as a leader?

When I was young, growing up in a war-torn country, I remember getting stuck on the interstate road with the bridges blown up behind me and in front of me. The soldiers were trying to clear the mines. I had a few days to get to the next city just 50 miles ahead to take an exam that would define my future. That night, I sat alone on the road and wondered whether I should break through the siege alone or wait with others until the road was cleared and miss my future.

Afterward, I was able to go to Germany for higher education and later to the US. I came to Stanley Fahn looking for a fellowship position. Reluctantly, Stan took me as a fellow and asked me to join the lab. We were trying to measure glycine in the brain and I was working to develop the technique based on a previous publication. I tried for more than a year without success. Finally, I called the author and learned that he had stopped the project because the techniques were unreliable. That night I sat wondering whether I should continue with my fellowship, trying to solve this problem, or look for something else and give up on an academic career.

A month later I was able to solve the problem. Stan gave me 6 test tubes to measure and when I returned with the results, he had a big smile on his face. This is the moment I am most proud of. Finally, I proved to him and to myself that I could be successful if I worked hard and was persistent.

What motivates you?

When I grew up, only 10% of our class was allowed to graduate. The ones who failed were drafted into the army, as we had a long war going on. I learned to be grateful for all the opportunities I was given, as many of my classmates did not even have this chance.

What steps do you take to resolve complicated leadership problems?

Many leadership problems are caused by misunderstanding, conflicting ambitions, and hypercompetitiveness. I try to delay my reactions to gain time to see where I can find common ground with others. Many years ago, I was advised to compartmentalize my feelings and the problem I was facing so that I could see it from a different angle and resolve the issue. I learned to focus on my objective and not be distracted by other people's actions.

In your mind, what are the main clues towards a successful career?

The main clue toward a successful career is to keep the long-term focus in your vision, together with the target date. If you know where you want to be 10 years from now, you will know where you have to be 5 years from now. If you know where you have to be 5 years from now, you will know where you have to be next year, and along with this, your next month's goal, tomorrow's target, and what you need to do in the next moment.

Chapter 42
VIDAILHET, Marie: Paris/France

Bios As a Neurologist, Movement Disorders doctor and clinical researcher, I had the opportunity to work with Pr. Yves Agid, in Salpêtriere University Hospital, both in clinic and in the research group in Paris, and in London, with Pr. David Marsden in Queen Square, two very inspiring and visionary scientists and neurologists, and with Pr Pierre Pollak, for deep brain stimulation in dystonia.

From the time I took the responsibility of the Neurology department, in Saint-Antoine University Hospital, Paris, we started a young movement disorders team that matured and expanded, during the next ten years, back in Salpêtriere hospital, Sorbonne Université. In the meantime, the research team was created in the ICM research Institute, and our focus is on pathophysiology and experimental therapeutics in dystonia and other movement disorders and in Parkinson's disease. In addition, I am actively involved in training and mentorship of Movement Disorders fellows (France, Europe and beyond) beside my implication in the Movement Disorders Society, and at the European level the MDS-ES section and the European Academy of Neurology (EAN).

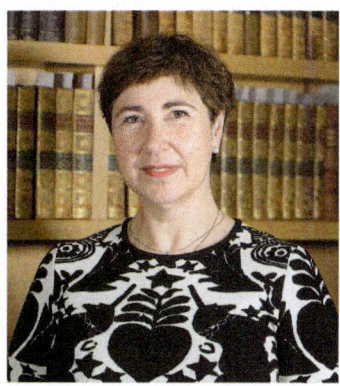

Reprinted with permission from Dr. Marie Vidailhet

M. Vidailhet (✉)
Department of Neurology, Salpetriere Hospital, AP-HP, Paris, France

Sorbonne Université, ICM UMR 1127, Inserm U 1127, CNRS UMR 7225, Paris, France
e-mail: marie.vidailhet@psl.aphp.fr

Did you ever consider leaving the career path you were on in order to doing something different (completely else or somewhat related)? What influenced you to stay and keep going?

Being a Movement Disorders doctor, and working with a team is a great privilege. I could not consider, looking back, leaving the career path and doing something different, even though I dreamed as a schoolgirl to be a cook, or an engineer to design planes or to build bridges. And indeed, building bridges between people, or between ideas is part of my daily life.

This is a great experience and a challenge to try, every day, to do my best, as a doctor and, if possible, as a person and to keep an open mind with creativity as a clinical researcher.

Team building is what fuels my energy: it is great to share knowledge, experience and enthusiasm with my peers and with young colleagues, so full of hope and energy. This is also a challenge, with joys and success and sometimes with difficult times, but this is what influences motto stay and keep me going.

Many people influenced me: my family gave me the sense of effort and duty, my friends energy and joy. With my colleagues, in the team, we trust each other and stand together: "one for all, all for one" is our motto! (this is of incredible value).

If you could go back and give your 21-year old self a valuable piece of advice, what would you say?

It is always hard to give a piece of advice that could be useful for everyone. But I would say: "Do your best, your very best, and do it over and over again, adapt to conditions and try to make them better, with solid work, generosity and fairness to people around you. This is a combination of dreams and projects, energy and pragmatism, sense of duty and independence. In any case, work hard and carry on!

This can be illustrated by a quotation from a French poet René Char. It is still in my office and can be translated as follows: "The impossible, we do not reach it, but it serves us as a lantern."

So my short piece of advice is: "believe in it, and do your best, always"

How would you track the performance of your team members and employees? How do you define and measure their success?

There are several ways to track the performances (although I do not like the formulation and would rather use the word "achievements" as it goes far beyond the concept of "performance".

First, there are milestones: medical and scientific knowledge, care with patients, staff, colleagues and juniors. This goes with the medical and academic degrees.

Each person has his/her optimal trajectory, there are slowly maturing people and fast runners! It is crucial to give everyone time.

Second, try not to choose the "best way" for the person but try to help him/her find what suits him/her best. This means guidance, interrogations and discussion and perspicacity to help people to see through their own projects and feelings and to decide what is their best path and commitment. This is, in my sense, what is mentorship.

Help people to give the best of their talents, to develop their strengths and to find fulfilment in their work without being too directive or too intrusive, is a challenge, and a heavy responsibility. This is a combination of self-initiative and team building spirit.

In one word, how do people define and measure their success: when they become better and more original and creative than their Mentor and are able to be inspirational to others.

How do you handle stress and pressures?

In our academic and medical work there is always some stress and pressure with bad days and good days. Hopefully good moments compensate for bad days, and a solid team does wonders: a person may have a different vision or the problem and another may have a solution to tackle the problem!! Stress and pressure are mainly related to my own work or responsibility. In order to relieve pressure at work, it helps to get back to a quiet office, to wash-out the worries and start with a fresh brain. Sometimes, it helps to go back to a simple duty, that is easy to do and perfectly mastered by experience. Or to spend all the energy to finish the job! Then enjoy the satisfaction of a job well done.

After work, stress and pressure can be relieved by reading a nice book, seeing friends and practicing my favorite sport activities or (French tradition) by cooking! Enjoy!

Chapter 43
YOUNG, Anne: Massachusetts/USA

Bios Anne B. Young Born December 30, 1947 in Evanston, Illinois. A.B. (chemistry) summa cum laude, Vassar College, 1969. M.D., 1973 and Ph.D. (Pharmacology), 1974, Johns Hopkins University School of Medicine. Intern in Medicine, Mt. Zion Hospital, San Francisco, 1975. Neurology Resident, University of California San Francisco, 1975–1978 (Chief Resident during final year). University of Michigan Neurology 1978–1991. Recruited to CHIEF OF NEUROLOGY, MASSACHUSETTS GENERAL HOSPITAL, 1991–2012; JULIEANNE DORN PROFESSOR OF NEUROLOGY, HARVARD MEDICAL SCHOOL, 1991—present. Member: Institute of Medicine; American Academy of Arts and Sciences; and the Royal College of Physicians (Fellow). She is the only person (male or female) to have been president of both the Society for Neuroscience (2003–2005) and the American Neurological Association (2001–2003). As a graduate student, Young provided the first biochemical evidence of glutamate as a neurotransmitter of the cerebellar granule cells. She developed biochemical techniques to measure inhibitory amino acid neurotransmitter receptors in mammalian brain and spinal cord. As a faculty member at the University of Michigan, Young and her late husband (John B. Penney, Jr.) worked together to establish the first biochemical data that glutamate was the neurotransmitter of the corticostriatal, corticobulbar and corticospinal pathways. They developed film-based techniques for quantitative receptor autoradiography. They also provided evidence for the most widely cited model of basal ganglia function (the basal ganglia are the brain regions affected by Huntington's and Parkinson's diseases). The model has provided the springboard for testing novel interventions in Huntington's and Parkinson's diseases and related disorders such as deep brain stimulation. Dr. Young was a key member of the US-Venezuela Huntington's disease Collaborative Research Project from 1981–2002 that found the HD gene and more. Dr. Young and her colleagues were the first to demonstrate gene expression changes in Huntington's and Parkinson's disease brains. Dr. Young established what is now called the MassGeneral Institute for Neurodegenerative Disease (MIND) in

A. B. Young (✉)
Harvard Medical School, Boston, MA, USA

Massachusetts General Hospital, Boston, MA, USA
e-mail: abyoung@partners.org

1999. MIND brings together scientists at MGH concentrating on studies of Alzheimer's, Parkinson's, Huntington's diseases and amyotrophic lateral sclerosis. Labs are encouraged to translate discoveries into assays for drug discovery and animal models for drug trials. Dr. Young spearheaded the comprehensive drug discovery efforts at the MIND and has been successful in identifying drug targets for Parkinson's, Huntington's and other neurodegenerative diseases.

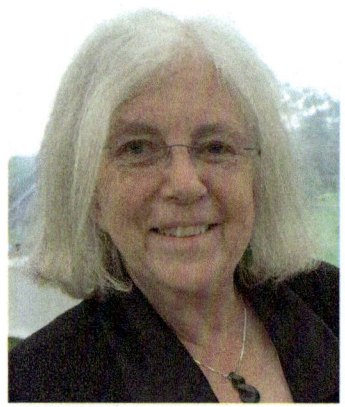

Reprinted with permission from Dr. Anne Young

What was the best advice you ever received in your early/late career?

Always get commitments in writing. I don't know who actually told me to get agreements in writing but doing so made important differences to me from medical and graduate school on. In medical school I designed my own MD/PhD program. I asked the medical school to allow me to spend all my elective time on my PhD. The Dean said 'yes' and I asked for it in writing. I asked the pharmacology department chair if he would allow my medical school courses to count for the PhD and he said 'yes' and I asked for it in writing. Both came in very handy in the end. After defending my thesis, the pharmacology department said they wanted me to stay another year because I was getting the two degrees in 5 years and it looked like Hopkins gave out cheap PhDs. I reminded them of the letters I had and how disappointed I was that they didn't stand by their commitments. They changed their minds the next day. Asking a chair or supervisor for a written offer is very standard but it is work for the chair and sometimes they leave out key items. You can always achieve your end by writing a return email saying you were so pleased to discuss a new position that would include blah, blah, blah.

Never come to your chair just asking for things. Always show your chair instead that by making a small commitment now will lead to a big return on investment.

Always arrange to control the minutes.
Always try to make deals that are win-win for everybody.

What are the challenges for a young scientist/academic/ clinician today compared to the past and how to tackle them?

The most challenging aspects for junior faculty today is that training is so long. Getting grants to cover salary and lab costs is more challenging now than in previous years. Fortunately many residencies now have research tracks that allow time in the lab during training. Also, this year the NIH budget has improved. Finally, trainees are more likely to be involved in big science than previously and therefore it is harder to become distinguished from others.

Can you share stories about mistakes, sometimes the best way to learn?

Early in my career, I had trouble controlling my temper. I blew up a number of times at people inappropriately and got into trouble. Learn to suppress your anger until you can have a calm discussion of the problem with the other person. Never put your angry feelings into writing. Take your time to put forth a calm response.

In your research there will be times when your experiments will turn out very differently than you predict. These observations often open up whole new ways of thinking about the problem and propel your research forward. Accept the findings and go for it!

Do you have advice addressed to young females in their early career?

Choose a partner who really wants to share all aspects of life together. Hire a great babysitter. If you have room for a live-in, that can be a big help for those with crazy schedules. For the lab, do your utmost to find the best person available to run your lab. Reward and promote that person so you can work together for your whole career.

Depression is common and most physicians won't admit their problems. Have a low bar for seeing a therapist. It can change your life.

Take an evening out once or twice a week.

The manufacturer's authorised representative in the EU is Springer Nature Customer Service Centre GmbH, Europaplatz 3, 69115 Heidelberg, Germany. If you have any concerns regarding our products, please contact ProductSafety@springernature.com

Printed and bound by CPI Group (UK) Ltd, Croydon, CR0 4YY

23/03/2026

02076444-0001